James Dunbar Dixon

History of Charles Dixon

One of the Early English Settlers of Sackville, N.B.

James Dunbar Dixon

History of Charles Dixon
One of the Early English Settlers of Sackville, N.B.

ISBN/EAN: 9783337326456

Printed in Europe, USA, Canada, Australia, Japan

Cover: Foto ©ninafisch / pixelio.de

More available books at **www.hansebooks.com**

HISTORY

—OF—

CHARLES DIXON,

—ONE OF THE—

Early English Settlers

—OF—

SACKVILLE, N. B.

COMPILED BY

JAMES D. DIXON,

A GRANDSON.

PRESS
FOREST CITY PUBLISHING CO.,
ROCKFORD, ILL., U. S. A.

PREFACE

THE object of the writer in compiling the within pages, is to give to the present and future generations some knowledge of their ancestry; and to put on record certain facts and events connected with their history, and as far as possible to record the names of the descendants of Charles Dixon down to the current year. To obtain the names of *all*, was found to be quite impracticable. The writer has personally visited numerous families, written scores and scores of letters, traveled hundreds of miles, and dilligently sought to obtain the information embodied in these pages; and while sincerely grateful for the measure of success attained, he deeply regrets that further greatly desired information respecting many of the families proved beyond his reach. For the errors and imperfections the work contains, he feels he may reasonably claim forbearance. The work has no claim or merit in a literary sense, the object sought being a simple, brief statement of facts and circumstances of little interest to any excepting the descendants of the aforesaid Charles Dixon. It was at first intended to bring the record down to the close of 1888, at which date some portion of the material had been collected. Circumstances, however, delayed the collection of the required information until a more recent period. Consequently it is probable many interesting events may have occured in connection with those families from whom he had obtained his information at the period first named, which are not recorded herein. To all who have aided him in his search for information, (who are too numerous to be recounted by name) his sincerest thanks are respectfully tendered. To the author of the History of the Black Family, who kindly gave him permission to use such portion of his account of the family of Martin G. and Fanny Smith Black as he might deem advisable, and which he has availed himself of to a certain extent, his acknowledgements are herewith tendered. In the hope that his effort to compile a family history extending over so many years and reaching the seventh generation and numbering nearly three thousand persons, may be duly appreciated and its many imperfections and errors regarded with much leniency, the compiler herewith dedicates his effort to the descendants of Charles and Susanna Dixon. J. D. D.

August, 1891.

N. B. The reader will observe that the figures prefixed to many of the names herein mentioned, are introduced for the purpose of indicating the Generation to which such persons belong, and their relationship to Charles and Susannah Dixon, who are accounted the *first* generation. Thus the figure 2 denotes the name is that of one of their children; the figure 3, one of their grandchildren; the figure 4, one of their great grandchildren, and so on.

HISTORY OF CHARLES DIXON, 1st.

CHAPTER I.

CHARLES DIXON came from Yorkshire, England, to Nova Scotia in the year 1772, and settled at Sackville, N. B. A paper written by himself, and dated Sept. 21st, 1773, giving some particulars of his life and history previous to that date, is herein transcribed, as follows:

I, Charles Dixon, was born March 8, old style, in the year 1730, at Kirleavington, near Yarm, in the East Riding of Yorkshire in Old England. I was brought up to the Bricklayer's trade with my Father until I was about nineteen years of age, and followed that calling till the 29th year of my age. I then engaged in a paper manufactory at Hutton Rudby, and followed that business for the space of about twelve years with success. At the age of thirty-one I married Susanna Coates, by whom I have had one son and four daughters. I was brought up a Protestant, or a member of the Church of England, and endeavored to demean myself as one on his Christian race; to live soberly, righteously and Godly in this present evil world, thinking, or at least had no doubt but I should obtain heaven at last. But being at one time at Robinhood's Bay, near Whitby, I went to hear Thomas

Secomb, a Methodist preacher, so called by way of derision. But his preaching was such as I never before heard, for his word was with power, it made me cry out in the bitterness of my soul, what must I do to be saved?

All my pretence of being a member of the church fell to the ground, I was condemned by her articles and homilies. I had broken my baptismal covenant, and was in fact a baptized heathen with a Christian name. For the space of about twelve months I went mourning all my days under a sense of guilt, and bowed down with the Spirit of bondage, but seeking for and asking of God, that Spirit wherewith He made His children free; that I might rejoice with his chosen, and give thanks with his inheritance. At length on Wednesday, September the 21st, 1765, while seeking and striving upon my knees, the Lord proclaimed his name merciful and gracious to forgive my iniquities, healed all my diseases, and set my soul at liberty. I was then a member of the Methodist Society at Hutton Rudby, and continued so till the year 1772, being the 42nd year of my age. Being wearied with public business, and I saw the troubles that were befalling my native country, oppressions of every kind abounded, and it was very difficult to earn bread, and keep a conscience void of offence, and though I was involved in business without the least appearance of being freed therefrom, until Providence so ordered it. The Honorable Lieutenant-Governor Franklin of the Province of Nova Scotia, at this time made some proposals for settlers; an acquaintance of mine, being his agent, with whom I had some intercourse. And when the advertisements came out I frequently recommended them to others, not seeing any way to embrace them myself, until about two months before I embarked at Liverpool. A gentleman I had never before seen called at my house and asked me some questions about my business, and told me that he was informed that I was inclined to embrace Governor Franklin's proposals, and if so he would undertake my business and purchase my stock and interest in Hutton Mills, that I might not be retarded. I was brought to think of it more seriously and gave him for answer that I would weigh it more narrowly, and give him a deliberate answer in a little time. After many thoughts, and consultations with my wife and friends, I came to a resolution to leave all my friends and interests I was invested with, and go to Nova Scotia. The time arrived that we were to be at Liverpool, and we reached there the 27th February, from whence we sailed on the 16th day of March, 1772, on board the Duke of York, with sixty-two souls, men, women and children, bound for Nova Scotia as settlers. My family consisted of myself, my wife and four children, viz: Mary, Charles, Susanna, and Elizabeth.

We had a rough passage, none of us having been at sea before; much sea sickness prevailed. After six weeks and four days, we arrived at Halifax, the capital of the Province, and were received with much joy by the gentlemen in general, but were much discouraged by others, and the account we heard of Cumberland (the place of our destination) was enough to make the stoutest heart give way. I had, however, an eye to that Providence that called and made things plain before me hitherto, and frequently told my wife all things would work together for good; not to be cast down, for I was sure we should meet with good success at our journey's end, and I endeavored to persuade others that He who had inclined us to come hither would surely not leave us, if we were not wanting to ourselves. Through many discouragements we arrived and landed at Fort Cumberland on the 21st day of May, and went into the Barracks with my family until we could find a resting place. At first glance things wore a very gloomy aspect. There were few of the inhabitants but wanted to sell their lands and go hence. I thought there must be some cause for this universal discontent. The spring was very late. I began to walk about the country, and went over to Sackville. After a few days investigation, finding the cause of discontent to be largely due to indolence and lack of knowledge, I purchased a tract of land at Sackville of Daniel Hawkins, containing 2500 acres, for the sum of £260. To which I removed my family on the 8th of June. Most of the rest of the settlers bought and settled elsewhere.

One thing in the inhabitants of Sackville at that time was very commendable; the not forsaking, but assembling together to worship, though unhappily divided into parties and ready to say to each other "I am holier than thou." And now let us admire that Providence which has preserved and brought us through many dangers from our Father's house and given us a lot in a strange land and an earthly inheritance that we never deserved or expected. Oh! that it may excite us to gratitude and thanksgiving while we dwell in a house of clay, and when this earthly tabernacle shall be dissolved may we receive an inheritance incorruptible, undefiled, that will never fade away; where the wicked will cease from troubling, and where our souls shall forever rest.

N. B.—This, my son Charles, is written for thy and thy little sisters' instruction, that thou be not high-minded, but

HISTORY OF CHARLES DIXON, 1st.

remember the rock from whence thou wast hewn, and in the future time when I and thy mother shall be called home, and rest in the silent grave, you may remember, that for your sakes we crossed the ocean. See that you outstrip us in purity of heart and holiness of life, and always let your words be the picture of your hearts. Study to adorn the doctrine and Gospel of God your Savior, and acquaint yourselves with God and be at peace. At peace with yourselves and with all men, and may the God of peace be with you evermore. Amen.

The following is also transcribed from a record made by the same person in his own hand-writing upon the flyleaf of his family bible: Sackville, N. B., 21st May, 1810. This day, 38 years ago, we landed at Fort Cumberland from Hutton Rudby, in Cleveland, Yorkshire, myself, my wife, Mary, Charles, Susanna and Elizabeth, six in all, and at this day the family has multiplied to ninety-four, all alive, save infants, and Ruth, my daughter, who departed 29th March last, much regretted by all who knew her, aged 37 years and three months, but our loss is her gain. She died as she lived, a Christian. Thus has the mercy and goodness of God followed us hitherto. (Signed,) CHARLES DIXON.

May 21st, 1815. This day, forty-three years ago, we landed at Fort Cumberland, with four children, viz: Mary, Charles, Susanna, and Elizabeth. Four more are added, viz: Ruth, Martha, Edward and William, all alive save a favorite, Ruth, and I suppose we are multiplied to not less, at this day than one hundred and thirty. But why are we thus multiplied and spared so long? Because God's mercy is over all his works. (Signed,) CHARLES DIXON. Aged 85.

HISTORY OF CHARLES DIXON, 1st.

The foregoing paper and records contain all that Mr. Dixon wrote respecting his own, or his family history. While the writer deems himself fortunate in the possession of these papers, he deeply regrets that Mr. Dixon did not leave on record some farther information respecting his parents, his brothers and sisters, and their families. He had a brother Edward, with whom he kept up a correspondence after coming to America, who also had a family. He for some time previous to his decease, was so afflicted with blindness, that he was obliged to employ some one to write his letters to his brother in America. There was also a sister, who was married to a Mr. Scotson, one of whose daughters married Abraham Bass, who was a tailor and draper of London, and who at Mr. Dixon's suggestion came to Sackville about the year 1810, and built a brick house on the site now occupied by the Chignecto Hall, where he kept a public house or hotel until his death. There was also John Dixon, an excise officer at Hutton Rudby, with whom Charles had business relations, while he was engaged in the manufacture of paper, who was probably a relative. There was also a Dixon family near the same locality, who at a later period gave to the Methodist church a distinguished minister, in the person of the Rev. James Dixon, D. D., who it is well known, in advanced age became totally blind. This latter circumstance coupled with the fact that a similar affliction existed in the case of Edward Dixon, before mentioned, and also with the fact that two of Charles Dixon's sons were in advanced age similarly afflicted, as will hereafter appear, tends to give color to the probability that the families had been nearly related in the not very remote past.

Charles Dixon very soon became an active and prominent

citizen of the community in which he had fixed his new home. He doubtless possessed some traits of character to be esteemed and admired. He was prompt in decision, firm of purpose, industrious, intelligent and conscientious in the discharge of his duties, and what his hand found to do, he did with his might. He possessed an education quite in advance of many of his associates and neighbors, and his twelve years' training in conducting the business of the paper mill had given him an aptitude for business, which would materially aid in qualifying him for efficiently discharging the duties of the positions he was so soon called upon to fill. He was called upon almost immediately to act as administrator of several Estates, among which was that of George Dobson, of Point De Bute, and one of Thomas Copple, of Petticodiac. He was also appointed a Justice of the peace in 1775, and Judge of the common pleas in 1778. As a Justice of the peace he had a large portion of the business of the Parish to perform for a lengthy period. He was also authorized to solemnize matrimony, and performed that duty for many of the early inhabitants.

Mr. Dixon was among the first of the English immigrants to what was then called Cumberland, Nova Scotia, (which included not only the present County of Cumberland, but also a large portion of the Province of New Brunswick, notably the counties of Westmoreland and Albert) who settled at Sackville, and believing that he had done wisely himself, he encouraged others of his Yorkshire acquaintance to follow his example; and when they arrived, aided them by his counsel, and in some instances with pecuniary assistance to enable them to make a start. What amount of funds Mr. Dixon brought from England is unknown, but beside the amount he paid for his land, he expended nearly as much in the purchase of stock of various kinds. He bought of Daniel Hawkins all *his* stock, consisting of horses, oxen, cows, young cattle and sheep. Of the latter he had more than a sufficiency, for he began immediately to lend them to his newly arrived acquaintances, to be returned, with their double in three years. As he still had funds to lend to his fellow immigrants, it is probable he was possessed of about a thousand pounds when he left England.

It would be interesting to know the names of the passengers with Charles Dixon, and his family, in the ship Duke of York. We are informed there were seventeen families, only one of which, so far as known, settled in Sackville beside Mr. Dixon. Thomas Anderson, with his wife Mary, who were married just previous to their departure from England, and who, after living for a year or so with Mr. Dixon, bought a a property on Coles' Island, of a Mr. Alvason, where they settled and became the founders of the extensive and respectable family of that name, many of whom are still residents of Sackville. William Freeze, and wife, and his wife's brother, George Bulmer, (who was a lad of twelve years) were also of the number of the same ship's company. Mr. Freeze first located at or near Amhurst, N. S., but finally settled at Sussex, Kings county, N. B., and became the founder of a numerous respected and influential family. George Bulmer, after completing his term of service with his brother-in-law Freeze, came to Sackville, purchased a property adjoining Mr. Dixon, and married into his family as will hereafter be seen.

For some years after Mr. Dixon came to Sackville he was engaged in a small way in merchandise, purchasing his goods and supplies, and marketing the surplus products of his farm at Halifax. This caused him to make occasional journeys to that city, going frequently by the way of Parrsboro and Windsor. On one occasion he met some old acquaintances in the persons of William and Jane Humphrey, who were then settled at Falmouth, N. S. Many years subsequently, after the death of Mr. Humphrey in 1795, Mr. Dixon advised Mrs. Humphrey to remove with her family of three sons and two daughters to Sackville, offering her a lot of his land situated on the main road through the village. Mrs. Humphrey accepted the offer promptly. A house was erected upon the lot, and in due time was occupied by herself and fanily. She was evidently a capable woman. She commenced very soon to keep a public house, so called, and her house was for many years a kind of headquarters where much of the semi-public or parish business was transacted. Mr. Dixon continued to hold his Justices courts there until within a brief period of his death. The place is now known as the farm of the late Christopher Humphrey.

Long previous to the removal of Mrs. Humphrey to Sackville, Mr. Dixon had encouraged John Richardson and his wife, whose maiden name was Mary Flintoff, and who was a sister of Mrs. Humphrey, to come to America, and who came out in the year 1774, and were then comfortably settled beside Mr. Dixon. One of Mr. Richardson's family was born on the ocean voyage, and was named Joseph Providence. The first name for the captain of the ship, and the second for the ship. John and Mary Richardson, above named, are the founders of the various families of that name in and around Sackville.

HISTORY OF CHARLES DIXON, 1st.

Very soon after the arrival of Mr. Dixon and the other English families who proce ded or immediately followed him, the Revolutionary War broke out. As a large proportion of the inhabitants of Sackville, at that period, were natives of Massachusetts, and the adjoining Colonies, and had only been absent from their native country a few years, it is not surprising that some of them should be inclined to sympathise with the Revolutionists, and actively espouse their cause; and aided and encouraged by a force from Calais they for a time beseiged Fort Cumberland. That enterprise however was soon abandoned, and they found more congenial employment in raiding the homes of the loyal and peaceable inhabitants, plundering them of such articles as they were in need of, and destroying or carrying away any guns or ammunition they might find. Mr. Dixon's home did not escape their unwelcome notice. His house was robbed of many valuable articles, some of which he kept for sale. For a considerable period the loyal inhabitants, notably the English settlers, were subjected to a state of anxiety, and lived in dread of a repetition of such unwelcome visits. On one occasion when some of these people were approaching the house, Mrs. Dixon hastily gathered up her silverware and other valuables and deposited them in a barrel of pig feed, where they quite escaped the notice of the visitors. On a later occasion, when somewhat similar troublous times existed, Mr. Dixon, with the aid of his negro servant Cleavelund, hid his money and other valuables in the earth; binding his servant by a solemn oath never to divulge to any one the place of concealment. These incidents may serve to remind us of some of the perils and difficulties our ancestors were compelled to encounter very soon after their arrival in the country.

At the close of the revolutionary war, the population of Nova Scotia was largely increased by the arrival of the Loyalists, many of whom settled at St. John and in that vicinity, and some came to Sackville, and others to Amherst and the adjacent localities. There was another class of persons who preceded the Loyalists, who came from the New England states, and some of whom settled at Sackville, who were termed refugees. These, it is understood, were not obliged to leave their native land because of their loyalty to the Crown and government of England. It can be truly said however, that the descendants of some of this class are now to be found among the most industrious and prosperous of our citizens.

Very soon after the close of the war, the Province of Nova Scotia was divided, and what is now known as the Province of New Brunswick was given a separate government.

An extract from the journals of the first session of the Legislature held at Parr Town, (now St. John) in January 1786, is here inserted and is as follows: "The consideration of the Sheriff's return for Westmoreland, being referred to a committee, the chairman reports, that the French votes are illegal, and that Charles Dixon was entitled to take his seat." And on February 7th, Charles Dixon appeared in the House, "And it was ordered that Mr. Hubbard and Mr. Paine, attend to see him qualified before the Commissioner for that purpose, who reported they had attended to that duty, and that Charles Dixon was duly qualified, and thereupon ordered that he take his seat."

Amos Botsford was the only other representative for the County until 1793, when four members were allowed to Westmoreland, and Amos Botsford, Thomas Chandler, William Black and Thomas Dickson were elected. Whether Mr. Dixon was a candidate for re-election in 1793 or otherwise the writer is not informed, nor does he know who beside Mr. Botsford and Mr. Dixon were the candidates at the first election. It is probable some other candidate had received more votes than he, including French, which when found to be illegal were stricken off, and Mr. Dixon became entitled to the seat. The revenue of the Province the first year was about £2500, out of which a grant was made to open a road to Westmoreland. The necessity for such grant was doubtless apparent by the fact that it required two weeks to inform Mr. Dixon of his right to the seat, and to enable him to appear at Parr Town.

Shortly after Mr. Dixon ceased to be a member of the Legislature he was appointed Collector of Customs and acted in that capacity some years. In the year 1788, he built a brick house, all the lumber for the floors and finishing of which was brought by water conveyance from the state of Maine. There was abundance of timber near at hand certainly, but the absence of mills for its manufacture no doubt necessitated that course. There is a building still standing owned by Mr. John E. Bowser, the boards of a portion of which also came from Maine at about the same time. A few lines of explanation in reference to the discontent which Mr. Dixon speaks of as being universal, may here be in order. After the expulsion of the French from Nova Scotia in 1755, efforts were made by the English authorities to induce persons living in the New England Colonies to come and occupy these vacant lands, and in

HISTORY OF CHARLES DIXON, 1st. 13

1758 and subsequently Governor Lawrence held out strong inducements which were to a certain extent successful. A Baptist church came *en masse* in the year 1763 and located at Sackville, other persons followed, and in the year 1765 the first grant of lands in Sackville was issued by the Government of Nova Scotia to these people, some of whom had served in the war against the French and were thus in part remunerated for such service. The whole parish of Sackville was thus granted and the holders of the said lands were the people to whom Mr. Dixon refers as being anxious to sell their lands and leave the country. The advent of the English immigrants who responded to Governor Franklin's proposals, and settled at Sackville, gave some of these people an opportunity to sell out and leave. At a later period when the Loyalists came others of them found opportunity to sell out to them, and others returned to their native country leaving their lands unsold.

Of the long list of persons whose names were contained in the original grants of Sackville, those who remained permanently are represented by the names of Ayr, Cole, Estabrooks, Kilham, Read, Tingley, Smith, Seaman and Ward.

The names of the English immigrants who settled at Sackville are Anderson, Atkinson, Bowser, Bulmer, Cornforth, Dixon, Fawcett, Harper, Patterson, Richardson and Wry. Most of whom were Methodists in their religious views. Those who settled at Point De Bute bore the names of Dobson, Chapman, Carter, Lowerison, Siddall, Trueman, Oulton, Trenholm, and others, many of whom were also Methodists, and others strongly attached to the Church of England.

Reference to Mr. Dixon's ledger supplies us with facts which though in harmony with the wants of society at that age, would be sadly at variance with present conditions. One or two of these may not be uninteresting. One entry shows that he hired a servant girl for the sum of nine pounds a year. And that one of the articles she required in payment for her services was a gallon of rum. Another shows that he purchased several negro slaves at Halifax, one of whom he sold to his friend, the Honorable Amos Botsford, at the same price he paid; another to his friend, Major Wilson, on similar terms, and one named Cleveland he retained for himself, for whom he paid the sum of sixty pounds, and to whom he subsequently gave his liberty, and thenceforth paid regular wages. This faithful old servant the writer can well recollect. He lived with Charles Dixon, Junior, after the death of his old master, and when dying, said he wished to be buried somewhere near his old master.

Mr. Dixon's house was a home for the early Methodist preachers, to whom he always gave a warm and hearty welcome. He was also one of the active members who erected the first Methodist church in Sackville, within whose walls he continued to worship until the infirmities of old age compelled his absence.

He, and his neighbor, William Cornforth, whose land adjoined, jointly set apart about four acres of land for a Methodist parsonage. A circumstance which had its influence in making Sackville the head of a circuit at that time. Previous to his death a brick house was erected on the lot so set apart, in the erection of which he also took a lively interest, and one of the latest of his efforts at writing contained instructions to his executors to sell certain articles of his personal property and apply the proceeds to assist in furnishing the parsonage.

It is proper that a few lines should be given to a notice of Mrs. Dixon, whose maiden name was Susanna Coates. But little is known with reference to her family. She was however a connection of an eminent thread manufacturing firm of that name in Manchester, and one of her younger sisters named Isabella, came to Nova Scotia about the same time she did, as the wife of John Trenholm. They settled at Point De Bute, and lived to advanced age, and were the progenitors of the numerous families of that name now living in Westmoreland and Cumberland and adjacent counties. The writer is of the opinion that the Coates family or families who came to Nova Scotia at about the same time Mr. Dixon came, and settled at Amherst and in King's county, were also relatives of Susanna and Isabel Coates. Mr. Dixon had quite extensive business relations with a William Coates for a number of years after he came to Sackville, and for whom he probably named his youngest son. Mrs. Dixon was blessed with a strong and vigorous constitution, and also in a marked degree possessed the ornament of a meek and quiet spirit. She cheerfully and patiently endured the discomforts and privations incident to pioneer life, while diligently discharging her duties as wife and mother. She was somewhat low in stature, though capable of an unusual amount of physical endurance. She was some nine years younger than her husband, but survived him as many years.

Mr. Dixon was a man of medium height, strongly built, and well proportioned, possessing an excellent constitution, capable of great physical exertion, and lived to ripe age. His death occured August 21st, 1817. Mrs. Dixon died June 13th, 1826. Each of them in the 88th year of their age. Near the site of the unpretentious church building which they and their co-laborers erected, and within whose walls they worshiped, their bodies lie buried; as do also many of the English immigrants before named, who were actively instrumental in founding Methodism in Sackville. As in life they lived and labored to promote a common object, in death they are not divided.

The family record of Charles Dixon as kept by himself here follows:

> Charles Dixon and Susannah Coates were married June 24th, 1763.
> Mary Dixon, born Friday, July 5, 1764.
> Charles Dixon, born Friday, January 10, 1766.
> Susannah Dixon, born Friday, July 24, 1767.
> Elizabeth Dixon, born Sunday, August 25, 1770.
> Ruth Dixon, born Wednesday, September 16, 1772.
> Martha Dixon, born Thursday, June 3, 1774.
> Edward Dixon, born Friday, September 20, 1776.
> William Coates Dixon, born Tuesday, February 23, 1779.

It will now be in order to trace out as far as practicable the genealogy of each of the above named persons, in their proper order. A chapter it will be observed is assigned to each.

GENEALOGY OF MARY DIXON AND HER HUSBAND WILLIAM CHAPMAN.

CHAPTER II.

²MARY DIXON, the eldest daughter of Charles and Susanna Dixon, married William Chapman, eldest son of William Chapman the 1st, who came to Nova Scotia in 1775 and settled at Point de Bute, and whose descendants are probably more numerous than any of the English immigrants of that period, and are scattered far and wide, although a host of the name still remains in the counties of Cumberland and Westmoreland.

William Chapman who married Mary Dixon in the year 1780, was a mechanic, who worked at the carpenter trade during the largest portion of his life. He did the joiner work of the brick house built by his father-in-law, Mr. Dixon, before mentioned. He settled at Fort Lawrence so called, where he had a valuable farm. The children of William Chapman and his wife, Mary Dixon, were:

William, born June 13, 1782. John, born Sept. 8, 1793.
Susanna, born March 19, 1784. Richard, born Sept. 8, 1795.
Elizabeth, born Feb'y 9, 1786. Jennie, born April 8, 1799.
Jane, born December 3, 1787. Sidney Smith, b'rn Aug. 13, 1801
Charles, born Sept. 28, 1789. Mary, born June 26, 1804.
Henry, born Sept. 2, 1791. Horatio Nelson, born — 1807.

2 Mary Dixon Chapman departed this life on the 22nd of December, 1837, in the 74th year of her age. Mr. Chapman survived his partner several years and died in March 1844, aged 87 years.

Mr. and Mrs. Chapman were honest, peaceable and industrious citizens, attendants upon the services of the Methodist church, within whose pale they found their spiritual home. Their remains rest in the Point de Bute Methodist church yard, which was a portion of the estate of the first Mr. Chapman, who gave it for a site for a Methodist church and burial place.

3 William Chapman, eldest son of William and Mary Dixon Chapman, about the year 1804 married Miss Harriet Bent. He also was a mechanic, as were very many of the Chapmans. He worked at ship carpenter work some considerable portion of his early life, and moved about to various places, residing at Sackville for a time and afterwards at Dorchester Island, from whence he went to Shepody so called, and finally settled at Salmon River, where he remained until his death. Their children were named Melvina, Eliza, Mary Ann, Clementina, John and Harriet. One or two others died in childhood.

Mr. and Mrs. Chapman died at Salmon River about the year 1870.

4 Melvina, the eldest daughter married a Mr. Martin, and they had some children, one of whom was Capt. Owen Martin, who died recently in Albert. Mrs. Martin removed to Boston, U. S., and if now living would be some 85 years of age.

4 Clementina, the fourth daughter of William and Harriet Chapman, married a Mr. Thomas Tingley, of Germantown Lake. Respecting the remaining members of this family no information has been obtained. It is probable they have re-

moved to the United States or have passed away from life many years since.

³ Susanna, eldest daughter of William and Mary Dixon Chapman, about the year 1820 married a Mr. John Greeno, of Newport, Nova Scotia. They settled at what is called the Chapman settlement, Cumberland county, where two of Mrs. Greeno's brothers settled about the same time, and which was then a dense wilderness. They had children named Mary Jane, William, John, Phoebe and Samuel. Mr. and Mrs. Greeno were thrifty, industrious people, and did much to redeem from the wilderness the village called the Chapman settlement. ³ Mrs. Greeno died in the year 1858, aged 73 years, and Mr. Greeno died in 1863, aged 64 years.

⁴ Mary Jane Greeno, eldest daughter of John and Susanna Chapman Greeno, married John Buchanan, a farmer, of Amherst Head, where they lived for some years and then removed to Lowell, Mass., with their family. Their children were named William, Susanna, John, James Wilson, Barbara, Samuel, Allen and Elizabeth.

Mr. Buchanan died in the year 1885, Mrs. Buchanan still survives. Their children are all dead except ⁵John, ⁵Allen and ₅ Elizabeth, who are married and some of whom have families.

⁴ William Greeno, eldest son of John and Susanna Chapman Greeno, married his cousin Miss Elizabeth Greeno, of Newport, Nova Scotia. They lived at Chapman Settlement, and followed farming. Their children are named, Leonard, Margaret, William, Susanna, Samuel, John, Allen, Rebecca, Frances and Florence.

⁴ William Greeno died in the year 1885, aged about 62: His widow still survives, residing at Chapman Settlement.

⁵ Leonard, eldest son of William and Elizabeth Greeno, married Annie E. Davis, of Northport, Cumberland county, N. S. He is a farmer and resides at Chapman Settlement, and has two children named James Edgar and Mabel.

⁵ Margaret, eldest daughter of William and Elizabeth Greeno, married Theodore Jackson, of Amherst. Mr. Jackson is an employe of the Inter-Colonial railway but owns a farm. Mr. and Mrs. Jackson had no family, and Mrs. Jackson died in the year 1882, aged 32 years. Mr. Jackson is again married to Sophia Hopkins and has a family.

⁵ William, the second son of William and Elizabeth Greeno, is married to Miss Sophia Burns, of Shinimicas, Nova Scotia, and resides there, farming. They have children named Laura, Lizzie, Walter and Maggie Bell.

⁵ Susanna, the second daughter of William and Elizabeth Greeno, married William Murray, a mechanic, of Pictou, Nova Scotia. They reside at Amherst. They have one child named Ethel Florence, and one other died in infancy.

⁵ Samuel, third son of William and Elizabeth Greeno, resides at Chapman Settlement, and follows farming, and is not married.

⁵ John, fourth son of William and Elizabeth Greeno, married Miss Ann Chapman, daughter of Howard Chapman, of Chapman Settlement, and resides at Northport, and follows lumbering. They have two children named Mary Blanche and Percy Blake.

⁵ Allen, the fifth son of William and Elizabeth Greeno, married Miss Sarah Jane Brooks, of Head of Amherst, where they reside, and follow farming. They have two children named Robert William and Russell Allen.

AND HER HUSBAND, WM. CHAPMAN.

⁵ Rebecca, third daughter of William and Elizabeth Greeno, married Frederic Brooks, a farmer, of Head of Amherst, where they reside, and have one child named Ralph.

⁵ Frances, fourth daughter of William and Elizabeth Greeno, married James Roach, son of Thomas Roach, of Amherst. They reside at Salem, and follow farming, and have no family.

⁵ Florence Greeno, youngest daughter of William and Elizabeth Greeno, died in 1883, aged 18 years, unmarried.

⁴ John Greeno, the second son of John and Susanna Chapman Greeno, married Miss Sarah Wells, daughter of Thomas Wells, of Point De Bute. They resided at Chapman Settlement, and followed farming. Their children were named Susanna, Dixon, John, Benjamin, Emma, Martha and Rufus, two others died in childhood. ⁴ Mr. John Greeno, died in 1875, aged 50 years. His widow still survives.

⁵ Susanna Greeno, eldest daughter of John and Sarah Wells Greeno, married Joshua Hatherly, of Minudie, N. S., a farmer; they reside at Amherst, farming, and have children named Edward, John, Irving, Leslie Allen and Bertha, four others died in infancy.

⁵ Dixon Greeno, eldest son of John and Sarah Wells Greeno, married a Miss Perkins, of Lowell, Mass. They reside in California, and have children named Frederic, George, Ralph and Cora.

⁵ John Greeno, the second son of John and Sarah Wells Greeno, married Miss Angeline Doyle, of Five Islands, where they reside and follow milling, &c. They have three children, one of whom is named Walter.

⁵ Benjamin Greeno, third son of John and Sarah Wells

Greeno, is a farmer, residing at Amherst Head, and unmarried.

[5] Emma and [5] Martha Greeno, daughters of John and Sarah Wells Greeno, died unmarried, aged 23 and 26 years respectively, as did also their brother [5] Rufus Greeno, aged 16 years.

[4] Phoebe Greeno, the second daughter of John and Susanna Chapman Greeno, married John Trenholm, a deputy sheriff, residing at Amherst. They had children named Amanda, Charles, Ellen, Clara, Sarah, Silas, James and Robert.

[4] Mrs. Trenholm died in 1878 aged 52 years. Her husband still survives.

[5] Amanda Trenholm, eldest daughter of John and Phoebe Greeno Trenholm, married John Bray, of New Glasgow, N. S., where they reside and are following mercantile pursuits. They have children named Walter, Ethel, Roy and others.

[5] Charles Trenholm resides near Lowell, Mass., and is not married.

[5] Ellen Trenholm, second daughter of John and Phoebe Greeno Trenholm, married William Cox, a shoemaker, and resides at Amherst. They had two children who died in infancy. Mrs. Cox died in 1879 aged 21 years.

[5] Clara Trenholm, third daughter of John and Phoebe Greeno Trenholm, married George Workman, a merchant, residing at Lawrence, Mass. They have one or more children.

[5] Sarah, fourth daughter of John and Phoebe Greeno Trenholm, is married to Edson B. Barnes, a farmer, residing at Winchenden, Mass.

[5] Silas and James Trenholm, sons of John and Phoebe Greeno Trenholm, also went to Massachusetts, where they still reside, unmarried.

⁵ Robert, youngest son of John and Phoebe Greeno Trenholm, resides at Amherst and is not married.

⁴ Samuel Greeno, the youngest son of John and Susanna Chapman Greeno, married Charity Wells, a daughter of Thomas Wells, of Point de Bute. They reside at Amherst Head, and follow farming, and had children named Thomas Wells, John William, Charles Wesley, Archibald H. and Samuel D. Mrs. Greeno died in 1864, at the age of 36 years, and ⁴ Mr. Greeno married Miss Lydia Wells, a sister of his first wife, and their children are named Robie, Erastus, Joseph Ernest and Courtland Roy, one other died in infancy, as did also an infant of the first wife's family. Mrs. Greeno, Samuel Greeno's second wife died in June 1888, aged fifty-one years. Mr. Greeno still survives.

⁵ Thomas Wells Greeno, eldest son of Samuel and Charity Wells Greeno, married Miss Eliza Nichols, of Vermont. They reside in Massachusetts and follow farming, and have one child named Mabel.

⁵ John William Greeno, second son of Samuel and Charity Wells Greeno, is a carpenter and resides in Massachusetts, where he married Miss Josephine Fleming. They have some family.

⁵ Charles Wesley Greeno, third son of Samuel and Charity Wells Greeno, is also in Massachusetts, engaged in farming, and is married.

⁵ Archibald H. Greeno, fourth son of Samuel and Charity Wells Greeno, married Miss Sophia Peers, who died in 1884, aged 22 years, leaving no children. Mr. Greeno then went to Rhode Island where he still resides, and is again married.

⁵ Samuel D. Greeno, youngest son of Samuel and Charity

Wells Greeno, married Miss Frances Wells and resides at Amherst Head and is farming. They have a child named Frederic Roland, and one died in childhood.

The second family of 4 Samuel Greeno are all at home and not married. This closes the history of Susanna Chapman, eldest daughter of Mary Dixon Chapman.

3 Elizabeth Chapman, the second daughter of William and Mary Dixon Chapman, married Nehemiah Ward, a farmer. They resided for a time at Buctouche, N. B., and then removed to or near Gagetown on the river St. John, where they lived for some years, then returned to Buctouche where they lived to advanced age. 3 Mrs. Ward died about the year 1860, aged about 75 years, and Mr. Ward a short time after. Their children were Mary Ann, Charles William D. C., Susanna, Fanny, Thomas, Nelson, Jane and Richard.

4 Mary Ann Ward, eldest daughter of Nehemiah and Elizabeth Chapman Ward, never married, and resided at St. John, N. B.

4 Charles William D. C. Ward, eldest son of Nehemiah and Elizabeth Chapman Ward, married Miss Catherine Ashley and resides at Buctouche and follows farming. Their children are named William N., James Edward, John Henry, Elizabeth Emerancy, Charles Pickard and Valentine Cutler. Four others died in childhood.

5 William N. Ward, eldest son of Charles W. D. C. and Catharine Ashley Ward, married Catharine Simpson, of Albert County, N. B. They reside at Buctouche and follow farming, and have children named Charles, Ada M., Thomas, Jane and Minor. Two others died in childhood.

5 James Edward Ward, second son of Charles W. D. C. and

Catharine Ashley Ward, married Miss Elsie Sears, of Sackville. They reside at Weldford, N. B., and follow farming. They have children named Delilah Edith, Fanny, Adelia, Mary Catharine, Elizabeth, Isaiah Dixon, Ella May and Maggie Graham.

6 Delilah Edith Ward, eldest daughter of James Edward and Elsie Sears Ward, is married to Henry Atkinson, of Weldford, where they reside. They have two children, James Robert and a babe.

The remaining children of 5 James Edward and Elsie Sears Ward are not married.

5 John Henry Ward, third son of Charles W. D. C. and Catharine Ashley Ward, married Miss Catharine McPherson, of Molus River, Kent Co., N. B. They reside at Newcastle, N. B. Mr. Ward is employed on the Intercolonial Railway. They have children named Wellington, Bertha, Mary Ann, Charles and two others.

5 Elizabeth Emerancey Ward, eldest daughter of Charles W. D. C. and Catharine Ashley Ward, married John Murray Ward, of Richibucto, N. B., and resides at Weldford, farming. Their children are named Alfred, Alma, Catharine, Charles, Ella Victoria and Julia.

5 Charles Pickard Ward, fourth son of Charles W. D. C. and Catharine Ashley Ward, married Miss Zilpha Estabrook, of Sackville, and resides at Buctouche, farming. Their children are Lillie May, Mary Ann, Chesley Melburn and Fanny Edith. One other died in infancy.

5 Valentine Cutler Ward, yongest son of Charles W. D. C. and Catharine Ashley Ward, married Miss Mary McDonald, of Buctouche, where they reside and follow farming. They have children named Milton, Frank and William.

⁴ Susanna Ward, second daughter of Nehemiah and Elizabeth Chapman Ward, died unmarried.

⁴ Fanny Ward, third daughter of Nehemiah and Elizabeth Chapman Ward, married Ichabod Pickett, of Belle Isle Bay, N. B. Their children were named Charles Peter, Mary Jane, Frances Ann, James Munson, Sarah Lavinia, Henry Wallace and Helen Louisa. After Mr. Pickett's death Mrs. Pickett married a Mr. Gunter, who is also dead, and Mrs. Gunter still survives.

⁵ Charles Peter Pickett, eldest son of Ichabod and Fanny Ward Pickett, is married but has no family.

⁵ Mary Jane Pickett, eldest daughter of Ichabod and Fanny Ward Pickett, married Charles Marvin, of Belle Isle, where they live. They had a daughter named Fanny, and a son. Mr. Marvin died about 1872.

⁵ Frances Ann Pickett, second daughter of Ichabod and Fanny Ward Pickett, is married and resides at Boston, Mass.

⁵ James Munson Pickett, second son of Ichabod and Fanny Ward Pickett, married a Miss Pickett. They reside in St. John, N. B.

⁵ Sarah Lavinia Pickett, third daughter of Ichabod and Fanny Ward Pickett, was married and died soon afterwards.

⁵ Henry Wallace Pickett, third son of Ichabod and Fanny Ward Pickett, married a Miss McLauchlan and resided at St. John. They had two children. Mr. Pickett is dead.

⁵ Helen Louisa Pickett, youngest daughter of Ichabod and Fanny Ward Pickett, married a Mr. Goslin, of Sussex, N. B. They reside at St. John.

⁴ Thomas Ward, second son of Nehemiah and Elizabeth Chapman Ward, married a Miss Trites, of Moncton, N. B.

They lived for a time at Buctouche, then removed to St. John. They have two daughters. Mr. Ward was killed by a man named Dowd, who was tried and executed for the crime a few years since. Mrs. Ward is also dead.

4 Nelson Ward, third son of Nehemiah and Elizabeth Chapman Ward, married Mary Wood, of Buctouche. They had two sons named Robert and John. Nelson Ward died some years ago, and his widow is still living.

5 Robert Ward, eldest son of Nelson and Mary Wood Ward, married a Miss Nellie Wood, of Machias, Maine. They reside in Massachusetts where Mr. Ward is a railway conductor, and they have some family.

5 John Ward, second son of Nelson and Mary Wood Ward, married Miss Jessie Seeley, of Cocaigne, N. B. They reside at Buctouche, and have children named Jane, Nelson, Fanny and Lulu.

4 Jane Ward fourth daughter of Nehemiah and Elizabeth Chapman Ward, married Robert Hyslop, a farmer, of Buctouche, where they resided. Their children are Ebenezer, Mary Ann, Melinda, and three others who died in childhood. 4 Mrs. Hyslop died in 1864. Mr. Hyslop is again married.

5 Ebenezer Hyslop, eldest son of Robert and Jane Ward Hyslop, married a Miss Burgess. They lived at Sussex, N. B., where he is employed on a railway. They had three children, one of whom is named Harry. Mrs. Hyslop died in 1890.

5 Mary Ann Hyslop, daughter of Robert and Jane Ward Hyslop, was a school teacher in St. John, and is married.

5 Melinda Hyslop, daughter of Robert and Jane Ward Hyslop, is also married.

4 Richard Ward, youngest son of Nehemiah and Elizabeth

Chapman Ward, married Jennie Tait, of Memramcook. They reside at Buctouche, farming. Their children are named Samuel, Henry, Mary Jane, Ida, Sarah Lavinia, Edgar, Murray Munson, Sylvester and two others who died in childhood. Two of the above named, [5] Samuel and [5] Mary Jane, also died in early life. The above is all that could be obtained respecting the posterity of [3] Elizabeth Chapman, and her husband, N. Ward.

[3] Jane Chapman, third daughter of William and Mary Dixon Chapman, married Andrew Weldon, of Dorchester. They resided at Buctouche, and followed farming. They had children named Elizabeth and John, and two others who died in childhood. [3] Mrs. Weldon died in 1826 aged 39 years. Mr. Weldon married for his second wife Mary Phinney. They had no family. Mr. Weldon died about 1870.

[4] Elizabeth Weldon, only daughter of Andrew and Jane Chapman Weldon, married James Atkinson, of Dorchester. They removed to Boston. They had children named Jane, David, Alice and two others.

[4] John Weldon, only son of Andrew and Jane Chapman Weldon, is a farmer residing at Buctouche. He married Miss Sarah A. Dickey, of Dorchester. Their children are Andrew, Charles Ovid, Julia Ann, Florence and Margaret. Three others died in childhood.

[5] Andrew Weldon, eldest son of John and Sarah A. Dickey Weldon, married Miss Crew. They reside in Boston, and have one child.

[5] Charles Ovid Weldon, second son of Andrew and Sarah A. Dickey Weldon, married Miss Mary Mugridge, of Shediac, N. B. They reside in Buctouche and follow farming. They have no family.

AND HER HUSBAND, WM. CHAPMAN.

5 Julia Ann Weldon, eldest daughter of John and Sarah A. Dickey Weldon, married Miles Farrell, a farmer, of Buctouche. Their children are named Ivy Maude, Luna and a babe not named.

5 Florence Weldon, second daughter of John and Sarah A. Dickey Weldon. married John McPhail, a farmer of Buctouche. Their children are named Charles, Sarah, Malcolm, William, Donald, Harry, Percival and John.

5 Margaret Weldon, youngest daughter of John and Sarah A. Dickey Weldon is not married. This closes the account of the posterity of 3 Jane Chapman and her husband, Andrew Weldon.

3 Charles Chapman, the second son of William and Mary Dixon Chapman, married Sarah Minard, of Parrsboro, N. S., where they resided. Mr. Chapman was a ship wright. Their family consisted of seven daughters and one son, viz: Amelia Elizabeth, Mary Jane, Ruth Roach, William Henry, Caroline, Margaret Sophia, Rebecca Eliza and Harriet Matilda. Mr. Chapman died in Parrsboro in 1848 aged 59. Mrs. Chapman died in 1876 aged 80.

4 Amelia E. Chapman, eldest daughter of Charles and Sarah Minard Chapman, married William Cook, a farmer, of Dorchester. They have no family. Mr. Cook died some years ago, and Mrs. Cook is still living.

4 Mary Jane Chapman, second daughter of Charles and Sarah Minard Chapman, was never married, and died many years since.

4 Ruth Roach Chapman, third daughter of Charles and Sarah Minard Chapman, married Hugh Ross. They resided at Parrsboro, and their children were named Elizabeth, Mary

Ann, Henry, Amelia and Sarah. Mrs. Ross died about 1878, and Mr. Ross is again married.

⁵ Elizabeth, eldest daughter of Hugh and Ruth Roach Chapman Ross, married a widower, the former husband of her youngest sister.

⁵ Mary Ann Ross, second daughter of Hugh and Ruth Roach Chapman Ross, died unmarried, aged 20 years.

⁵ Henry Ross and ⁵ Amelia Ross are not married.

⁵ Sarah Ross, the youngest daughter of Hugh and Ruth Roach Chapman Ross, married and had one child, and died soon after. Her husband married her eldest sister as before stated.

⁴ William Henry and ⁴ Harriet Matilda Chapman, children of Charles and Sarah Minnard Chapman, died in early life.

⁴ Caroline Chapman, fourth daugnter of Charles and Sarah Minnard Chapman, married John Minnard, of Upper Brookfield, a farmer. They had several children, when Mrs. Minnard died and her husband married again.

⁴ Margaret Sophia Chapman, fifth daughter of Charles and Sarah Minnard Chapman, married Ainsley Steeves, a prominent mechanic of Amherst, where they reside. Their children are named William, Julia A., Laura S. and Minnie. Four others died in infancy.

⁵ William Steeves, only son of Ainsley and Margaret S. Chapman Steeves, married Miss Sarah Frazer, of Pictou. They resided at Amherst and had four children named Winnie, Percy, Birdie and Reta. Mr. Steeves died in October, 1884, aged 31 years. He was an excellent mechanic. His widow and family reside at Amherst.

⁵ Julia A. Steeves, eldest daughter of Ainsley and Margaret S. Chapman Steeves, is unmarried and resides with her parents.

⁵ Laura Steeves, second daughter of Ainsley and Margaret S. Chapman Steeves, married William Redpath, a mechanic of Boston, Mass., where they reside. They had three children, all of whom died in childhood.

⁵ Minnie Steeves, the youngest daughter of Ainsley and Margaret S. Chapman Steeves, married William Wallace, a mechanic of Sussex, N. B., where they reside and have one son named George Stanley. Another child died in infancy.

⁴ Rebecca Eliza Chapman, sixth daughter of Charles and Sarah Minnard Chapman, married a Mr. Bishop, of Albert County, N. B., where they reside.

The above closes the account of the posterity of ³ Charles Chapman.

³ Henry Chapman, third son of William and Mary Dixon Chapman, married Isabel Jones, of Point de Bute, and soon afterward, with his brother John Chapman and his brother-in-law John Greeno, removed to what now is called the Chapman Settlement, then a dense wilderness. It is stated that William Chapman, father of the above named Henry and John, who lived at Fort Lawrence, with some of his associates who were fond of the sport, used occasionally to go moose hunting, and sometimes visited the locality above mentioned, and near a meadow there which bore a heavy burden of wild grass, that noble animal was frequently found and killed. Mr. Chapman made application to Government and procured a grant of a large block of land in the vicinity where he subsequently settled his sons before mentioned. The meadows yielded these pioneers of the forest a supply of hay for their stock, which the almost entire absence of roads for several years and their

great distance from the marshes would have made it difficult to procure otherwise.

The children of Henry and Isabel Jones Chapman were named George, Fanny, Henry, Sidney, Susan Jane, William, Richard, Martin and Howard. Mrs. Isabel Chapman died in 1837, aged 39 years. Mr. Henry Chapman married a second wife, a Mrs. Martha Trenholm. The issue of this marriage was one daughter named Ellen Adelia. [3] Mr. Chapman died in 1869, aged 68 years. His widow survived several years.

[4] George Chapman, eldest son of Henry and Isabel Jones Chapman, married Barbara Buchanan. They resided at Chapman Settlement, farming. Their children are named Martha, Isabella, Rebecca, Sarah Jane, Woodford Henry, Alexander Clark, Frances, Janet, Arthur and Martha, and another who died in infancy.

[5] Martha and [5] Isabella, the two eldest of the above named children of George and Barbara B. Chapman, died unmarried, each of them at the age of 20 years.

[5] Rebecca, the third daughter of George and Barbara B. Chapman, married Charles Hill, a farmer, residing on the Tindal road, so called. Their children are named Hattie, Lewis and George.

[5] Sarah Jane, fourth daughter of George and Barbara B. Chapman, married Harmon Bent, farmer, of Salem, Cumberland Co., N. S., and their children are named George, Alonzo and Gaius.

[5] Woodford Henry, eldest son of George and Barbara B. Chapman, when a young man, was lost in the Gulf of Mexico when on his first voyage at sea, in the year 1872.

[5] Alexander Clark, second son of George and Barbara B.

AND HER HUSBAND, WM. CHAPMAN.   33

Chapman, married his cousin, Mary Ellen, daughter of Henry and Sarah Lowther Chapman. They lived at Head of Amherst and followed farming. Their children are Walter Stanley, Clark Bishop and Arthur Raymond. Mrs. Chapman died in the year 1887, aged 34 years. Mr. Alexander Clark Chapman is again married to Miss Jane Beharrell, of Head of Amherst.

5 Frances, the fifth daughter of George and Barbara B. Chapman, is not married and resides at Lowell, Mass.

5 Janet, sixth daughter of George and Barbara B. Chapman, is married to Willis Baxter, of Head of Amherst. Their children are George, Frances, Carl and a babe.

5 Arthur, third son of George and Barbara B. Chapman, is a mechanic and resides at Minneapolis, Minn., and is married.

5 Martha, youngest daughter of George and Barbara B. Chapman, married Herbert Atkinson, a farmer, son of Gilbert Atkinson Esq., of Amherst. Their children are named Roy and Ivy Venola.

4 Fanny, the eldest daughter of Henry and Isabel Jones Chapman, married Charles D. Rockwell, of Amherst Shore, a farmer and mechanic. They had one son named James Henry. Mrs. Rockwell died in 1842, aged 22 years. Mr. Rockwell is married again to a Miss Perrigo, and has a family.

5 James Henry, only son of Charles D. and Fanny Chapman Rockwell, married Mary Boultenhouse, of Bathurst, N. B. They reside at River Herbert, N. S. Mr. Rockwell is a superior mechanic. Their children are named Charles, Avard, Joseph, Laura, Mary and Edith. Three others died in childhood.

4 Henry, second son of Henry and Isabel Jones Chapman,

married Miss Sarah Lowther. He is a farmer, and resides at Chapman Settlement, upon the homestead of his father. Their children are named Caroline, Frances, Joseph Henry, Martha, Isabel, Esther, William S. Darragh, Mary Ellen, Moses, Ezra, Alice, Sarah and Thomas. Mrs. Chapman died in the year 1865, aged 48 years. Mr. Chapman is married again to a sister of his first wife, Miss Emmeline Lowther. The names of the children of the second family are Celia, Cora, Charlotte, Rebecca, Agnes, Robert, Cecil, Joshua, Garnet P., Stephen P. and Tudor Grace.

[5] Caroline, eldest daughter of Henry and Sarah Lowther Chapman, married Mr. Isaac Beharrell, a wealthy and prosperous farmer, of Amherst. They have children named Elizabeth, Mary and Ada.

[5] Frances, second daughter of Henry and Sarah Lowther Chapman, married Edmund Doyle, of Tidnish River, where they resided and were engaged in farming and lumbering. Their children are named Edith, Frances and William, the two last named being twins. Two others died in infancy. Mrs. Doyle died in 1879, aged 36 years. Mr. Doyle is married again to Miss Jane Irving.

[5] Joseph Henry, the eldest son of Henry and Sarah Lowther Chapman, was for some years a seafaring man, and sailed on foreign voyages. He resides at Amherst, and is known by the title of Captain Chapman. He married a German lady, Miss Agnes Rhor, of Bremerhaven. Their children are named Henry Theodore, Agnes, Lewis, Fretia, Olga and a babe. One other died in infancy.

[5] Martha, third daughter of Henry and Sarah Lowther Chapman, married Frank Mason, a farmer, at Head of Am-

herst. Their children are John Wilbur, Guy Earlscott, Stevely Gee and five others who died in infancy and childhood.

⁵ Isabel, the fourth daughter of Henry and Sarah Lowther Chapman, is not married and resides at Lowell, Mass.

⁵ Esther, fifth daughter of Henry and Sarah Lowther Chapman, married Thomas Davis, a farmer, residing at Bayside, N. B. Their children are Henry, Garfield, Mary, Mabel and Edith.

⁵ William S. Darragh, second son of Henry and Sarah Lowther Chapman, married Miss Letitia Read, of Vermont, U. S., and resides at Lowell, Mass. He is a carpenter. They have a child named Freddie.

⁵ Mary Ellen, sixth daughter of Henry and Sarah Lowther Chapman, married Alexander Clark Chapman as before stated.

⁵ Moses, third son of Henry and Sarah Lowther Chapman, married Sarah Jane Allen, of Bayside, N. B., and resides at Chapman Settlement, farming. Their children are Allen, Hattie and Frances.

⁵ Ezra, the fourth son of Henry and Sarah Lowther Chapman, is not married, residing in Boston, Mass.

⁵ Alice, seventh daughter of Henry and Sarah Lowther Chapman, is married to Elisha Webber, a farmer residing at Bowdoinham, Maine. They have one child named Susan.

⁵ Sarah, the eighth daughter of Henry and Sarah Lowther Chapman, is not married and resides for the most part at Lowell, Mass.

⁵ Thomas, fifth son of Henry and Sarah Lowther Chapman, is a mechanic, residing in Brookfield, Mass. Not married.

The family of ⁴ Henry Chapman by his second wife Emmeline Lowther Chapman, are not married, residing at home with their parents.

⁴ Sidney, the third son of Henry and Isabel Jones Chapman, married Miss Ellen Horton, a daughter of James and Elizabeth Keillor Horton. They settled at Chapman Settlement, and have reclaimed from the wilderness a large farm, where they still reside. Their family consists of six sons and three daughters, named George Joel, Joseph Ripley, Martha Elizabeth, Frances Isabel, James Henry, Hannah Melinda, Thomas Sidney, Martin Bedford and Woodford Edgar, one other died in infancy.

⁵ George Joel, eldest son of Sidney and Ellen Horton Chapman, is a ship carpenter, and for a number of years followed that occupation in various portions of the United States. He has a farm at Mt. Pleasant near Oxford, Nova Scotia, where he now resides, unmarried.

⁵ Joseph Ripley, second son of Sidney and Ellen Horton Chapman, is not married. He lives at Vancouver, British Columbia, and follows farming and lumbering.

⁵ Martha Elizabeth, eldest daughter of Sidney and Ellen Horton Chapman, married George Patterson, of Amherst, and they now reside at Richmond, Maine. They have one child named Flora Bell. Mr. Patterson is engaged in lumbering.

⁵ Frances Isabel, second daughter of Sidney and Ellen Horton Chapman, married Bradford Bowlsby, a carpenter, of Londonderry, N. S. They reside at Maccan, N. S., and have children named Lillian May, Chester Elmore, Al aretta, Zdisque Lovell, Ellen Rebecca, Ada and Eva.

⁵ James Henry, third son of Sidney and Ellen Horton Chapman, married Mary Oulton, daughter of Charles Oulton,

Esq., and reside at Mt. Pleasant, near Oxford, N. S., farming. They have one child named Mabel Edna.

⁵ Hannah Melinda, third daughter of Sidney and Ellen Horton Chapman, married Mr. Chapman Gooden, of Coburg, Westmoreland, N. B., where they reside and follow farming. They have children named Wilson, Melvina, Sidney Chapman, and Ora Hester.

⁵ Thomas Sidney, fourth son of Sidney and Ellen Horton Chapman, married Miss Frederica A. Rolph, of Shediac, N. B. They reside at Mt. Pleasant, N. S., and follow farming. They have children named Frank Frederic, Clarence Bradford and Ernest Sidney.

⁵ Martin Bedford, fifth, and ⁵ Woodford Edgar, sixth, sons of Sidney and Ellen Horton Chapman, are yet unmarried, and reside at home with their parents.

⁴ Susan Jane, the second daughter of Henry and Isabel Jones Chapman, married Stephen Peacock, a farmer of Botsford Parish, N. B., where they resided. Their children were named Henry Chapman, Cordelia Elizabeth, Mary Jane, Job Seaman, Margaret Isabel, Hannah Ann, Rebecca Frances, Stephen Lee and Solomon Boyd. Mr. Peacock died in the year 1881, aged sixty-two years, and Mrs. Peacock died in 1882, aged fifty-three years.

⁵ Henry Chapman Peacock, eldest son of Stephen and Susan Jane Chapman Peacock, married Elizabeth Jane Blacklock. They resided at Botsford and have children named William Clark, Stephen Arthur and Frances. Mr. Peacock follows farming and milling.

⁵ Cordelia Elizabeth Peacock, eldest daughter of Stephen and Susan Jane Chapman Peacock, married Nelson Anderson,

a farmer of Botsford, where they reside. Their children are named Stephen Boyd, Phoebe Hannah, William Henry and Susan Jane.

⁵ Mary Jane Peacock, second daughter of Stephen and Susan Jane Chapman Peacock, married William Blacklock, a farmer of Botsford, and their children are named Mary Elizabeth and Albert. One other died in childhood.

⁵ Job Seaman Peacock, second son of Stephen and Susan Jane Chapman Peacock, married Miss Jane Welch, of Botsford. They reside at Botsford, farming, and have children named Fletcher, Jane and Susan Chapman.

⁵ Margaret Isabel Peacock, third daughter of Stephen and Susan Jane Chapman Peacock, married Robert Lamb, a farmer of Botsford, where they reside and have one child named Janet Maria.

⁵ Hannah Ann Peacock, fourth daughter of Stephen and Susan Jane Chapman Peacock, married William A. Scott, a farmer of Botsford. They have one child named Ella Rebecca.

⁵ Rebecca Frances Peacock, fifth daughter of Stephen and Susan Jane Chapman Peacock, is not married, and resides at Botsford with her brother Solomon.

⁵ Stephen Lee Peacock, third son of Stephen and Susan Jane Chapman Peacock, is a school teacher residing at Botsford and is not married.

⁵ Solomon Boyd Peacock, youngest son of Stephen and Susan Jane Chapman Peacock, is a farmer residing upon his father's farm in Botsford with his sister Rebecca Frances, and is not married.

⁴ William Chapman, the fourth son of Henry and Isabel Jones Chapman, married Miss Jane Finley, of Head of Am-

herst, and resides at Chapman Settlement and is farming. Their children are James Henry Coats, Esther Isabel, Maggie Jane, Edwin Ruthven, Emma Mabel, Boyd Thomson, Joseph Johnson, Mary Laura, George Ephraim and Martin Call.

[5] James Henry Coats, the eldest son of William and Jane Finley Chapman, is not married and resides at home with his parents.

[5] Esther Isabel, the eldest daughter of William and Jane Finley Chapman, married William H. Chapman, of Port Elgin, N. B., where they reside and have one child named Lorne.

[5] Maggie Jane, second daughter of William and Jane Finley Chapman, married James A. Chapman, a farmer of Port Elgin, N. B., where they reside, and have children named Albert Floyd and Maggie Lizzie.

[5] Edwin Ruthven, second son of William and Jane Finley Chapman, is a shoemaker residing in Boston, Mass., and is not married.

[5] Emma Mabel, third daughter of William and Jane Finley Chapman, married William Ainsley Chapman, a farmer residing at Chapman Settlement. Their children are named Wallace Lee and Maynard Rene.

[5] Mary Laura, fourth daughter of William and Jane Finley Chapman, is married to Andrew Olsen, a farmer residing at Linden. N. S.

The remaining children of William and Jane Finley Chapman are not married and reside with their parents.

[4] Richard Chapman, fifth son of Henry and Isabel Jones Chapman, married Catherine Wells, a daughter of William Wells, of Point de Bute. They reside at Head of Amherst and follow farming. Their children are named Susan Jane, Abi-

gail Rebecca, Margaret Ellen, William Henry, George Thomson, Joseph Elmore, Lillie Maud and Frank Wilbur; one other died in childhood.

⁴ Richard Chapman died in 1887, aged 54 years. His widow still survives and resides at Head of Amherst.

⁵ Susan Jane, eldest daughter of Richard and Catherine Wells Chapman, married Oscar Melvin. They reside at Los Angelos, Cal. No family.

⁵ Abigail Rebecca, third daughter of Richard and Catherine Wells Chapman, married Charles Watson, electrician, residing at Nashua, New Hampshire. They have one child named Neva Maud.

⁵ Margaret Ellen, third daughter of Richard and Catherine Wells Chapman, married William Barrett, a farmer of Tidnish. They had one child named Margaret Etta. Mrs. Barrett died in 1884, aged 22 years.

⁵ William Henry, eldest son of Richard and Catherine Wells Chapman, married Miss Emmeline Chapman, daughter of Howard Chapman, of Chapman settlement. They reside at Head of Amherst, farming.

⁵ George Thomson, second son of Richard and Catherine Wells Chapman, is not married, and resides at Nashua, New Hampshire, and is employed in the electric light works.

⁵ Joseph Elmore, ⁵ Lillie Maud and ⁵ Frank Wilbur, the remaining children of Richard and Catherine Wells Chapman, are at home with their mother and not married.

⁴ Martin Chapman, the sixth son of Henry and Isabel Jones Chapman, was never married, and died at the age of 22 years.

⁴ Howard Chapman, the seventh and youngest son of

Henry and Isabel Jones Chapman, is married and resides at Spring Hill Mines, N. S. They have children, one of whom is named George.

⁴ Ellen Adelia, only daughter of Henry Chapman and Martha Trenholm, married Gilbert P., only son of John Black, of Amherst. They had two children who died in infancy. Mrs. Black also died in the year 1862, when about 22 years of age. This closes the account of the posterity of Henry Chapman and his wife Isabel Jones, and his second wife Martha Trenholm.

³ John Chapman, fourth son of William and Mary Dixon Chapman, married Miss Jane Jonah in the year 1817. They settled at Chapman Settlement, as stated on a former page, and very largely assisted in redeeming from the wilderness the now flourishing settlement of that name. What hardships and privations those pioneer settlers endured, without roads for many years, except blazed pathways through the wilderness which were impassable except on foot or on horseback, and far distant from any other settlement, can now be only faintly appreciated or understood. The two brothers, Henry and John Chapman, and their brother-in-law John Greeno, bravely battled with and overcame all obstacles confronting them in their persistent attempt to carve out for themselves productive farms and comfortable homes. The success which crowned their efforts is now seen in the flourishing village before mentioned, principally occupied by their descendants. The children of John and his wife Jane Jonah Chapman, were named William, George, Ann, John, Ruth, Henry, Silas, James, Edmund, Elizabeth, Howard, Hiram, Wesley and Sylvanus; one other died in childhood. John Chapman and his wife Jane both died in 1883, aged 90 and 85 years respectively.

[4] William, eldest son of John and Jane Jonah Chapman, married Margaret Riley, of Shemogue, N. B. They reside at Chapman Settlement, farming. Their children are named Almond, James, John Cooper, Mary Jane, Margery and Lucius Mickey.

[5] Almond, eldest son of William and Margaret Riley Chapman, resides at Port Elgin, and follows milling.

[5] James, the second son of William and Margaret Riley Chapman, married a widow lady, Mrs. Annie Carson. They live at Sussex, N. B., and have one child named Margaret Hattie.

[5] John Cooper, third son of William and Margaret Riley Chapman, married Miss Alice Morrison of Amherst Shore. They reside at Gray's Road near Oxford, N. S. They have one child named Sanford W. Daniel.

[5] Mary Jane, eldest daughter of William and Margaret Riley Chapman, married Mortimer Smith of Shinimicas; he is a mill man and resides at Chapman Settlement. They have children named Oliver Walter, Ruby Jane, John M., Ray R. Arlington and William Norman. Two others died in childhood.

[5] Margery, second daughter of William and Margaret Riley Chapman, married Thomas Ogden, a farmer of Chapman Settlement. They have one child named Lucius Melbourne.

[5] Lucius Mickey, youngest son of William and Margaret Riley Chapman, married Miss Alice L. Ogden, and resides at Chapman Settlement and follows farming.

[4] George, the second son of John and Jane Jonah Chapman, married Catherine Roberts of Amherst. They lived at Chapman Settlement, and had one child which died in childhood. George Chapman is supposed to have been drowned in

crossing the Straits from Prince Edward Island in a small vessel, which was lost with all on board. He was 25 years of age when the sad event occurred in the year 1845. Mrs. Chapman afterward married Mr. Milner Purdy of Amherst.

4 Ann, eldest daughter of John and Jane Jonah Chapman, married Weldon Jackson, a farmer of Amherst Shore, where she now resides. Their children are named Elizabeth A., Leonard S., James J., Jane, and John H. Mr. Jackson died in the year 1885, aged 65 years.

5 Elizabeth A., eldest daughter of Weldon and Ann Chapman Jackson, married Charles Fields, a farmer. They reside at Amherst Shore, and their children are named Ernest Alton, Leonard Purdis, Ora Leonora and Lauretta Violet.

5 Leonard S., eldest son of Weldon and Ann Chapman Jackson, died unmarried in 1880, aged 30 years.

5 James J., second son of Weldon and Ann Chapman Jackson, was drowned in the year 1878, aged 26 years. He was not married.

5 Jane, second daughter of Weldon and Ann Chapman Jackson, resides at Lowell, Mass.

5 John H., youngest son of Weldon and Ann Chapman Jackson, resides at home with his mother, and follows farming.

4 John Chapman, third son of John and Jane Jonah Chapman, married Miss Lillie Riley. He resided at Port Elgin, N. B., and followed farming and milling. Their children are George, James A., William Hiram, John Douglas and two others who died in childhood. Mr. Chapman died in 1875, aged 50. His widow survives.

5 George, the oldest son of John and Lillie Riley Chapman, married Miss Elizabeth Gooden, of Port Elgin, and lives at

Chapman Settlement, and follows milling. They have children named Barbara and Isabella.

⁵ James A., second son of John and Lillie Riley Chapman, married Miss Maggie Jane Chapman, daughter of William and Jane Finley Chapman, as stated on page 39.

⁵ William Hiram, third son of John and Lillie Riley Chapman, married Esther Isabel, daughter of William and Jane Finley Chapman, of Chapman Settlement, as stated on page 39.

⁵ John Douglas, youngest son of John and Lillie Riley Chapman, resides at Port Elgin and follows milling.

⁴ Ruth, second daughter of John and Jane Jonah Chapman, married William Riley, a farmer. They lived at Chapman Settlement, and had children named James, Margaret, Hiram and Barbara. Mr. Riley died in 1860 at the age of 40 years, and Mrs. Riley died in 1887, aged 62 years.

⁵ James, eldest son of William and Ruth Chapman Riley, went to British Columbia, where he was engaged in hunting and mining. He is married.

⁵ Margaret, eldest daughter of William and Ruth Chapman Riley, married James Stephens, a farmer residing near Spring Hill, N. S.

⁵ Hiram, second son of William and Ruth Chapman Riley, is a miner residing at Spring Hill. He married a Miss Smith. They have children, one of whom is named William.

⁵ Barbara, youngest daughter of William and Ruth Chapman Riley, resides in Boston, dressmaking.

⁴ Henry, fourth son of John and Jane Jonah Chapman, married Miss Diana Smith, of Shinimicas. They lived at Chapman Settlement, and followed farming. Their children are named Harvey, Jane, Hibbert, Abigail, Iintha and Lavinia

Victoria. Mrs. Chapman died in 1867, aged 35 years. Mr. Chapman married Miss Jane Brownell for his second wife. They had one child named Henry Dearborn. Mr. Chapman and his family removed from Nova Scotia many years ago, and when last heard from lived in the state of Maine.

⁵ Harvey, the eldest son of Henry and Diana Smith Chapman, is married and has some family.

⁵ Jane, the eldest daughter of Henry and Diana Smith Chapman, is married to a Mr. Smith, of Maine, and has some family.

⁵ Lavinia Victoria, youngest daughter of Henry and Diana Smith Chapman, is likewise married and has some family.

⁴ Silas, the fifth son of John and Jane Jonah Chapman, married Miss Eliza Jones, of Newport, N. S. He was a millright, and lived for a time at Chapman Settlement, but subsequently removed to Newport, the home of his wife. They had children named Ira, George W., Ida Jane, Catharine, Celestia, Everite, Minnie, James Kenneth, Herbert and Cyrus Maxwell, Mr. Silas Chapman died in 1876, aged 45 years. His widow married Bazilla Lake, and resides at Brooklyn, Newport, N. S.

⁵ Ira, eldest son of Silas and Eliza Jones Chapman, married Miss Emma Hues, of Ellerhouse. He is a millright. They reside at Windsor Forks, N. S., and have children named Charles, William, Mabel and Edward.

⁵ George N., second son of Silas and Eliza Jones Chapman, married Miss Ellen Best, of St. Croix, N. S. He is a harnessmaker and resides at Brooklyn; they have two children named George R. and James H., two others died in childhood.

⁵ Ida Jane, eldest daughter of Silas and Eliza Jones Chap-

man, married Herbert Riley, of St. Croix. They had a child named Morton, and another who died in infancy. Mr. Riley also died, and Mrs. Riley married Mr. Archibald Robinson, of Windsor, and they have a child named Ruby, and another a babe.

[5] Catharine, second daughter of Silas and Eliza Jones Chapman, married John White, a painter, of Brooklyn, N. S. They had two children named John and Eva. Mrs. White died in 1883, in the 21st year of her age.

[5] Celestia, third daughter of Silas and Eliza Jones Chapman, married Frank Cole, of Lynn, Mass., where they reside, and have a child named Lucy.

[5] Everite, [5] James Kenneth, [5] Herbert, [5] Minnie and [5] Cyrus Maxwell, are all unmarried. The last named being at home with his mother, and the others in Lynn, Mass.

[4] James, sixth son of John and Jane Jonah Chapman, married Mary Low, daughter of Anthony Low, of Amherst Shore, They resided for a time at Chapman Settlement, farming, and had children named Charles, Amelia, Andrew, Emma, James A., Arthur and two others. They removed to Winnipeg some years ago with most of their family, where they still reside.

[5] Amelia, the eldest daughter of James and Mary Low Chapman, married Melville Bird, of Athol, N. S., where they reside and have several children.

[5] Andrew, the second son of James and Mary Low Chapman, died in 1868, aged 10 years.

[4] Edward, the seventh son of John and Jane Jonah Chapman, is a carpenter at Chapman Settlement, and is not married.

⁴ Elizabeth, third daughter of John and Jane Jonah Chapman, married George Hayward, a farmer and millman, residing at Woodside, N. B. Their children are Silas, Ephraim, Jane, Aramatilda, Clara and one other, who died in childhood.

⁵ Silas, eldest son of George and Elizabeth Chapman Hayward, married Miss Mary Louisa Tingley, and resides at Port Elgin, N. B. They have children named Florence, Athelwood, Elmore and Charles Tupper.

⁵ Ephraim, second son of George and Elizabeth Chapman Hayward, married Mary Black, of Richibucto. They reside at Woodside, N. B., and have children named George Nelson, Bruce LeBaron and James Harvey.

⁵ Aramatilda, second daughter of George and Elizabeth Chapman Hayward, is residing in Nevada, unmarried.

⁵ Jane and Clara, the eldest and youngest daughters of George and Elizabeth Chapman Hayward, reside at home with their parents, unmarried.

⁴ Howard, eighth son of John and Jane Jonah Chapman, married Elizabeth Ogden, of Amherst Shore, and resides at Chapman Settlement, occupied in farming and lumbering. Their children are Annie M., Jane, Howard D., Willard, Emmeline, Rosilla, Isadora, Hazen, George, Ruby, Sarah, Dusit and Harold.

⁵ Annie M. eldest daughter of Howard and Elizabeth Ogden Chapman, is married to John Greeno, son of Wm. Greeno. See history of Greeno family.

⁵ Jane, second daughter of Howard and Elizabeth Ogden Chapman, is not married and resides in Boston, Mass.

⁵ Howard D., eldest son of Howard and Elizabeth Ogden

Chapman, is married to Susan Chapman, of Tidnish River, and lives at Chapman Settlement, farming.

[5] Willard, second son of Howard and Elizabeth Ogden Chapman, is not married, and resides at home, farming.

[5] Emmeline, third daughter of Howard and Elizabeth Ogden Chapman, is married to William Henry Chapman, of Head of Amherst. See page 40.

[5] Rosilla, fourth daughter of Howard and Elizabeth Ogden Chapman is not married, and resides in Boston with her sister Jane.

The remaining members of the family of Howard and Elizabeth Ogden Chapman, are at home with their parents, unmarried.

[4] Hiram, ninth son of John and Jane Jonah Chapman, married Sarah M. Ogden, of Amherst Shore, and resides at Chapman Settlement on the homestead farm of his father. He is a farmer and is also largely engaged in lumbering, and owns a steam saw mill which he personally superintends. Their children are named William Ainsley, Victoria M., Ellen L., Amanda A., Joseph E., Udivella M., Charles M., Sanford W., John W., Hiram Leslie, Leonard O. and Annie E. Two others died in childhood.

[5] William Ainsley, eldest son of Hiram and Sarah M. Ogden Chapman, is married to Emma M. Chapman, daughter of William and Jane Finley Chapman, as stated on page 39.

[5] Victoria M., eldest daughter of Hiram and Sarah M. Ogden Chapman, married William Tweedy McKay, and resided at Chapman Settlement. They had two children who died in childhood. Mr. McKay died in the year 1885, aged 26. Mrs. McKay is living at Chapman Settlement.

⁵ Ellen L., Second daughter of Hiram and Sarah M. Ogden Chapman, is married to Joseph Gallant, a mechanic of East Boston, where they reside. They had one child who died in infancy. The remaining children of Hiram and Sarah M. Ogden Chapman are unmarried.

⁴ Wesley, tenth son of John and Jane Jonah Chapman, married Charlotte Jane Graham, and resided at Bay du Vin, Northumberland Co,, N. B., where he followed the occupation of a miller. They had one child named William. Wesley Chapman died in 1875, aged 32 years. His widow afterward married a Mr. Kerr.

⁴ Sylvanus, youngest son of John and Jane Jonah Chapman, married Miss Adeline Smith, daughter of Thomas R. Smith, of Shinimicas. Sylvanus is a blacksmith and lives at Shinimicas. Their children are George, Ella Jane, Mary Ann, Ivan and a babe.

This closes the account of the posterity of John and Jane Jonah Chapman.

³ Richard Chapman, fifth son of William and Mary Dixon Chapman, married Jane Wells, daughter of William Wells of Point de Bute, N. B., and resided for a number of years on the homestead farm of his father at Fort Lawrence, and followed farming. He subsequently removed to Head of Amherst or Chapman Settlement, where he followed farming until his death, in the year 1872, at the age of 77 years. His widow still survives. Their children are named, William Wells, Elizabeth Augusta, Richard Wesley, and Henry Walsten.

⁴ William Wells, eldest son of Richard and Jane Wells Chapman, married Mary A. Beharrell, and resides at Amherst Head, farming. Their children are named Udivella, William Wallace,

George Botsford, Clara Amelia, Archibald Clarence, Alma Rebecca, Robert Stewart, Maggie Jane, Frank, Eva Bell and two who died in infancy and childhood.

5 Udivella, eldest daughter of William Wells and Mary A. Beharrell Chapman is married to a Mr. Joseph G. Lake. They reside in Boston, Mass. The remainder of the family of William Wells and Mary A. Beharrell Chapman are unmarried.

4 Elizabeth Augusta, only daughter of Richard and Jane Wells Chapman, died in 1853, aged 15 years.

4 Richard Wesley, second son of Richard and Jane Wells Chapman, married Sarah Jane Wells of Head of Amherst. They reside at Beecham Settlement, farming, and have children named Charles Wesley, Emma Jane, Olivia, Etta, Mary Eliza, Thomas Melzar, Arabella, and Henry Walsten, four others died in infancy.

5 Charles Wesley, eldest son of Richard Wesley and Sarah Jane Wells Chapman, married Miss Amelia Bird, of Athol, Cumberland county, N. S. They reside at Beecham settlement, farming, and have one child, a babe.

5 Emma Jane, eldest daughter of Richard Wesley and Sarah J. Wells Chapman, is married to George S. Robinson, carriage maker at Tidnish cross-roads, and they have two children, Hertha Bell and a babe. The remainder of the family of Richard Wesley and Sarah J. Wells Chapman are unmarried and at home.

4 Henry Walsten, youngest son of Richard and Jane Wells Chapman, married Miss Olivia Brundage, daughter of Thompson Brundage, of Tidnish. Their children are named Richard Thompson, Ella Mabel, James Percy, Etta Maud, Georgiana, Henry Walsten and Ada; one other died in childhood. 4 Henry

Walsten Chapman is a superior mechanic and resides at Moncton, and has a good situation in the Government Railway Works. The children are all at home with their parents. This closes the account of the posterity of Richard and Jane Wells Chapman.

3 Jennie, daughter of William and Mary Dixon Chapman, died in childhood from the effects of eating some poisonous plant.

3 Sidney Smith Chapman, sixth son of William and Mary Dixon Chapman, married Miss Elizabeth Kay, of Buctouche. They resided there and followed farming and other occupations. Their children were named Mary, James Kay, Margaret Weldon, Jane, Thomas, William Wesley, Samuel Dwight, Allison Edmonson, Sarah Elizabeth, Robert Ainsley and Hannah Emmeline. 3 Sidney Smith Chapman died in 1864, aged 63 years, and Mrs. Chapman died 1869, aged 64.

4 Mary, the eldest daughter of Sidney S. and Elizabeth Kay Chapman, died at the age of 30 years, unmarried.

4 James Kay, eldest son of Sidney Smith and Elizabeth Kay Chapman, married Susan Coster, of Tidnish, N. S. They lived at Buctouche, N. B., and had one child, named Charles Chapman. Mr. Chapman was a mechanic. He died in 1886, aged 50. Mrs. Chapman died in 1870, aged 29.

5 Charles Chapman, son of James Kay and Susan Coster Chapman, is not married and resides at Moncton, N. B.

4 Margaret Weldon, second daughter of Sidney S. and Elizabeth Kay Chapman, married William Crossman, farmer, of Shemogue, where they resided. They had no family, and Mrs. Crossman died in 1860, aged 30 years.

4 Jane, third daughter of Sidney S. and Elizabeth Kay

Chapman, married Jeremiah Marshman, a seafaring man of Buctouche. They had children, named Gladys, Richard and Emma. Mrs. Marshman died in 1884, aged 52 years. Her husband still survives.

⁵ Gladys, eldest daughter of Jeremiah and Jane Chapman Marshman, married John Hawes, a carpenter of Moncton, and died soon after her marriage; and after some time Mr. Hawes married ⁵ Emma Marshman, sister of his first wife.

⁵ Richard Marshman is unmarried and resides at Moncton.

⁴ Thomas, second son of Sidney S. and Elizabeth Kay Chapman, married Miss Louisa C. Chappell, of Tidnish, daughter of Liffey Chappell. Mr. Thomas Chapman is an excellent mechanic, and resides at Tidnish. The children are named Albion Jane, Lillia Dale, Susan Rayworth, Oscar Fitzallen, Alexander Tuttle, Alfred Ernest, Almira Louisa and Edna Florence. Mrs. Chapman died July 11, 1881, aged 45 years.

⁵ Albion Jane, eldest daughter of Thomas and Louisa C. Chappell Chapman, married Anderson Trenholm, of Tidnish, a farmer. Their children are Susan Gertrude, and a babe.

⁵ Lillia Dale, second daughter of Thomas and Louisa C. Chappell Chapman, married Arthur Barratt, of Tidnish. They had children, named Agnes Georgiana and Louisa Caroline. Mr. Barratt died in 1885, aged 26 years. His widow survives, residing at Tidnish.

⁵ Susan Rayworth, third daughter of Thomas and Louisa C. Chappell Chapman, married Howard D. Chapman, eldest son of Howard Chapman, of Chapman Settlement, as before stated on page 47. The other children of Thomas and Louisa C. Chappell Chapman are at home, unmarried.

⁴ William Wesley, third son of Sidney S. and Elizabeth

Kay Chapman, married Miss Sarah Morrison, of Buctouche. He followed the coasting business for some time, but now resides at Moncton, and is employed in the Government Railway Works. Their children are named Elizabeth Jane, William, Ella, Ida, John, Harry Wesley and Mary Alice, all unmarried.

4 Samuel Dwight, fourth son of Sidney S. and Elizabeth Kay Chapman, married Miss Jane Cutler, and lived for a time in Picton county, N. S. They have no family.

4 Allison Edmonson, fifth son of Sidney S. and Elizabeth Kay Chapman, when a young man went to the United States, and it is said was for a time during the war of the rebellion in the U. S. Navy. When last heard from he was in Florida, unmarried.

4 Sarah Elizabeth, fourth daughter of Sidney S. and Elizabeth Kay Chapman, married Mr. James Cameron, a farmer, of Buctouche, where they still reside. Their children are named Frederic Barnesby, Hannah Abigail, William James, Amanda Jane, Robert, John Sidney, Elizabeth Kay, Charles Edward and a babe; none of whom are married.

4 Robert Ainsley, sixth son of Sidney S. and Elizabeth Kay Chapman, married Miss Margaret Price, of Moncton, where they reside. Their children are Elizabeth Tyle, William Leslie, John Sidney, Dimock, Annie Cora, Clinton Purdy and one who died in infancy. Mr. Robert Ainsley Chapman is a mechanic.

4 Hannah Emmeline, youngest daughter of Sidney S. and Elizabeth Kay Chapman, died unmarried in 1879, aged 27 years. This closes the account of the posterity of Sidney Smith Chapman and his wife Elizabeth K. Chapman.

³ Mary, the youngest daughter of William and Mary Dixon Chapman, married Luke Doyle, a shipwright. They resided principally at Amherst, and their children were named James, John, Catharine, Martin and Benjamin. Mrs. Doyle died in 1887, aged 83 years. Mr. Doyle still survives.

⁴ James, the eldest son of Luke and Mary Chapman Doyle, went to Lowell, Mass., many years ago, and is said to be married and to have several children.

⁴ John, second son of Luke and Mary Chapman Doyle, died in 1861, aged 24 years. He was not married.

₄ Catharine Doyle, only daughter of Luke and Mary Chapman Doyle, married James Hicks, a farmer, of Buctouche, where they resided until the death of Mr. Hicks, who died in 1884, aged 48 years. They have children, named Ira, Lewis, Rebecca, Manford, Maria, Prudence, Fanny, Catharine and Silas. Mrs. Hicks, after the death of her husband, removed with her family to Moncton, where she still resides.

⁵ Ira, the eldest son of James and Catharine Doyle Hicks, went to the United States when a young man and was last heard of at Calais, Maine.

⁵ Lewis, second son of James and Catharine Doyle Hicks, married a Miss Jones, and resides at Moncton and is employed on the railway.

⁵ Fanny, the fourth daughter of James and Catharine Doyle Hicks, married Albert Lyons, of Shediac, where they reside. He is employed on the railway. They have one child, an infant. All the remainder of the family of James and Catharine Doyle Hicks are unmarried and reside at Moncton, except ⁵ Maria, who lives at St. John, N. B.

4 Martin, third son of Luke and Mary Chapman Doyle, died unmarried.

4 Benjamin, youngest son of Luke and Mary Chapman Doyle, resides in Amherst. He married a widow lady named Goldsmith, and their family consists of John E. Mary E. Hanse Masters, Emma Jane and Rena Bell. Seven others died in childhood. The children above named are all at home with their parents. This closes the account of the posterity of Mary Chapman and her husband Luke Doyle.

3 Horatio Nelson, the youngest son of William and Mary Dixon Chapman, when considerably advanced in years married a Miss Woodworth daughter of Charles Woodworth, formerly of Sackville. They resided for a time in Westmoreland and also at Fort Lawrence, and had children named Charles, Lucy, Henry and others whose names have not been ascertained. 3 Mr. Chapman and his family all went to the United States many years ago. The author has failed to procure the address of any of this family and therefore is unable to give reliable information respecting them. It is said that 4 Henry married a woman of some property in Maine, and that 4 Lucy married a man by the name of Stackhouse. 3 Mr. Chapman, if living, which is scarcely probable, would be about 84 years old.

Here closes the history of the posterity of Mary Dixon, and her husband William Chapman.

The following statement of the posterity of Mary Dixon and her husband William Chapman is compiled from the foregoing records, and from careful estimates of the numbers of the descendants of some the branches, concerning whom positive information could not be obtained.

GENEALOGY OF MARY DIXON.

	Born.	Living.	Dead.
Children	12	0	12
Grand "	85	45	40
Great Grand "	393	303	90
Great Great Grand "	360	293	67
Great Great Great Grand "	4	4	
Total	854	645	209

GENEALOGY OF CHARLES DIXON, SECOND.

CHAPTER III.

[2] CHARLES DIXON, eldest son of Charles and Susanna Coates Dixon, was six years old when he left England and came with his parents to Nova Scotia. He was a healthy, vigorous youth, capable of any amount of physical endurance. At the age of sixteen, during the closing years of the revolutionary war, he, with other youths of Sackville and vicinity, was taken to Fort Cumberland to perform garrison duty, and acquitted themselves creditably.

In the year 1788 he married Miss Rhoda Emmerson, a daughter of one of the original grantees of Sackville. At the same hour of the same day and in the same house, Miss Martha Grace was married to Ebenezer Cole. In their family were included the late Michael Grace Cole, Rufus Cole, Esq., and Capt. Martin Cole, all of whom were well known residents of Sackville.

[2] Mr. Dixon settled on a portion of the land purchased by his father of Daniel Hawkins and rapidly redeemed the same from the wilderness and turned it into fruitful fields. The children of Charles and Rhoda Emmerson Dixon were:

William, born August 7, 1789.
Charles, born March 22, 1791. (Died in infancy.)
Charles, born June 8, 1793.
Hannah, born September 6, 1795.
Benjamin, born December 18, 1797.

Mrs. Rhoda E. Dixon died July 27, 1799, in the thirtieth year of her age. Mr. Dixon soon after married Miss Elizabeth Humphrey, eldest daughter of Mrs. William Humphrey, of whom mention has been previously made. This marriage occurring so soon after the death of his first wife so shocked the sense of propriety of Mr. Dixon's Methodist associates (for he was a member of the Methodist Society) as to cause for a time some estrangement. His parents, however, were the more inclined to overlook the offence, inasmuch as the bride being a Yorkshire Lass the alliance was regarded by them with more favor than the former one. Doubtless they believed as most Yorkshire people do to the present day, that there is no one quite the equal of a good Yorkshireman.

² Charles Dixon and Elizabeth Humphrey were married 13th of October, 1799. Their children are:—

John, born August 9, 1800.
Sidney, born Aug./5, 1805.
Jane, born Oct. 13, 1810.
Christopher Flintoff, May 6, 1816.
Alfred, born January 31, 1821.
Elizabeth, born January 1, 1803.
Leonard, born July 12, 1808.
Ruth, born August 4, 1813.
Edward, born August 17, 1818.
Mary, born July 13, 1823.
Martha, born June 27, 1825.

² Mr. Dixon turned his attention occasionally to various enterprises quite outside of his farming operations. He also had a strong desire to see some other portions of America. And about the year 1803, he with a young man, a neighbor, named Timothy Richardson, visited the United States, through which they journeyed, much of the time on foot, until they reached Ohio, and at or near the place now called Cincinnati they had a boat constructed in which they pursued

their journey to New Orleans. From thence they took passage by sea to New York, where in due time they arrived. Mr. Dixon, however, fell ill with fever and ague which occasioned increased expenses and delay. Fortunately his brother-in-law, George Bulmer, was in the city, and finding them out rendered them such pecuniary aid as they required to enable them to pursue their journey homeward. They then took passage for home with one Capt. Burnham, and at Mount Desert they were detained by the severity of the weather for a considerable time, but at length reached home in safety. Whether Mr. Dixon or his companion then had thoughts of finding a home in the United States, is not known. Soon after his return home he made preparations for brewing ale, and erected one or two stone buildings for that purpose, near where the residence of J. R. Rainie now stands. This enterprise not proving a success, he next turned his attention to the erection of a windmill near the same spot. This also proved unsuccessful, and he subsequently made extensive preparations, and built another mill on a much more expensive scale which stood near his own residence. This one promised to give good satisfaction but was unfortunately destroyed by fire and proved a serious pecuniary loss. In 1825 he with his son-in-law Mr. McKinlay, entered into an arrangement to build a ship, upon which in the early part of 1826 they had made considerable progress, when news came from England of a serious decline in the price of ships. They then ceased work, and about two years subsequently sold out to other parties who completed the vessel. After this unprofitable speculation Mr. Dixon confined his attention quite successfully to his farm until he sold out, and removed with his wife and seven youngest children to Ohio in the year 1837. Mr. Dixon's removal to Ohio was due to the fact, that he and several of his family had recently embraced the views of the people called Mormons, or Latter day Saints, and he felt it to be the only safe and proper course for him to pursue. The writer has a vivid recollection of an interview that took place between Mr. Dixon and his brother Edward, at which he earnestly pressed upon his brother's consideration, his recently embraced views, and faithfully exhorted him to follow his example, and warning him of the folly and danger of remaining in a country so soon to be destroyed as he believed.

[2] Mr. Dixon and family left Sackville on the first day of September. 1837, and traveled in a number of covered wagons, arriving at Kirtland, Ohio, the place of their destination, on the 14th of October, where he purchased a property and settled his family. The year following in the autumn, he, with his daughter Jane and youngest son, started for Missouri. Soon after they had crossed the Missouri River they met large numbers of the Mormon people, who were being driven out of that State by force, most of whom were in a most destitute condition. They returned with these people to Quincy, Ill., where Mr. Dixon hired a house and remained for the winter, and liberally used his means in entertaining and relieving the necessities of these poor suffering, destitute brethren. The following spring he returned to Ohio, where he pursued with his usual diligence and industry his occupation of farming, until the spring of 1854. When he had entered upon his 89th year, and had become nearly blind, he and his wife, with some of the family, left Ohio for Salt Lake City. They arrived at Rock Island and halted for a few days, while their party were

fitting up and getting their teams ready for the journey across the plains. Here, Mr. Dixon, on account of his blindness, fell from the steps of a hotel and sustained injuries which proved fatal, and his death occurred on the 22d day of May. He was buried at Davenport, Iowa. The family pursued their journey, arriving safely at their destination. Mrs. Dixon survived her husband some eleven years and died at about the same age.

3 William, eldest son of Charles and Rhoda Emmerson Dixon, married Elizabeth Weldon, daughter of Andrew Weldon, Esq., of Dorchester. They settled at Memramcook, where he followed farming and milling. Their children were named Andrew, Charles, Rhoda, John Weldon, William, Edward, Amasa and Elizabeth Ann.

3 William Dixon, died in the year 1830, aged 40 years. His widow afterward married a Mr. Evans, a cabinet maker. They had two children, and Mrs. Evans died in 1854, aged 60 years.

4 Andrew, the eldest son of William and Elizabeth Weldon Dixon, was a mechanic, and for some years in company with his brother Charles, carried on carriage building at Dorchester. He was not married, and died in 1848, aged 35 years.

4 Charles, second son of William and Elizabeth Dixon, is also a mechanic and has continued to reside at Dorchester, pursuing his occupation. His wife was a Mrs. Flynn. and their children are named Frank, Charles, William, Andy, Annie and Arthur and Arthur, all of whom are unmarried.

4 Rhoda, eldest daughter of William and Elizabeth Weldon Dixon, married John Budd, who resided at Westchester, N. S., farming. Their children are William Dixon, Jacob

Purdy, James and Mary Jane. Mr. Budd died in 1885. His widow still survives.

⁵ William D., eldest son of John and Rhoda Dixon Budd, married a Miss Allen. They lived at Five Islands, N. S., and followed farming. Mr. Budd died some years since, leaving a widow and several children.

⁴ John W., third son of William and Elizabeth Weldon Dixon, was also a mechanic, and engaged in the manufacture of leather, shoes, and harness at Dorchester. He married Miss Mary C. Stiles, daughter of Enoch Stiles, Esq., and their children are named Celia Elizabeth, William, Bertha, and John W. ⁴ Mr. Dixon was killed while raising the frame of a barn, a part of which accidentally fell, striking his head. His sudden and lamented death occurred in 1853, in the 35th year of his age. His widow survived many years and died in 1880.

⁵ Celia Elizabeth, eldest daughter of John W., and Mary C. Stiles Dixon, married John T. Dickie, a manufacturer and ship owner of Dorchester, and they have a family, named Scott Hutton, Myrtle, Mabel, and John, none of whom are married.

⁵ William, eldest son of John W., and Mary C. Stiles Dixon, is a deaf mute, and was educated at the Institute for deaf mutes at Halixax, N. S. He is a superior mechanic, resides at Dorchester and is not married.

⁵ Bertha second daughter of John W. and Mary C. Stiles Dixon, married Captain Charles Anderson of Sackville. They have children named George, Rheese, Calista, Bertha and Pearl. Captain Anderson and his family now reside in New Zealand.

⁵ John W. youngest son of John W. and Mary C. Stiles

GENEALOGY OF CHARLES DIXON, 2D.   63

Dixon, was lost at sea in 1873. The vessel in which he sailed not being heard of after leaving Dorchester.

⁴ William, fourth son of William and Elizabeth Weldon Dixon, married Jane, youngest daughter of John Chapman, Esq. of Dorchester. They resided at Dorchester, where Mr. Dixon carried on a carriage factory for many years. Their children are Sophronia, William Chipman, Sophia Gertrude and Humphrey Pickard. Two others died in infancy. Mr. Dixon died in 1890, aged 69 years. His widow still survives.

⁵ Sophronia, eldest daughter of William and Jane Chapman Dixon married Robert A. Colpitts, Merchant of Dorchester, they have no family.

⁵ William Chipman, eldest son of William and Jane Chapman Dixon, died at the age of eighteen years.

₅ Sophia Gertrude, second daughter of William and Jane Chapman, Dixon, married Captain Herbert Chambers, Shipmaster. They have children named Harry Colpitt and Roy Chapman. Mrs. Chambers resides at her mother's home in Dorchester while her husband is at sea.

⁵ Humphrey Pickard, youngest son of William and Jane Chapman Dixon, is a mechanic and sometimes follows seafaring, and is not married.

⁴ Edward, fifth son of William and Elizabeth Weldon Dixon, was also a mechanic and engaged in the shoemaking business at Napan, N. S., where he married a widow lady who was a daughter of Gaius Lewis, Esq., of Parrsboro, N. S. This marriage took place in 1848. They had children named Amasa, Eunice, Mary Emma and Amelia A. Mr. Dixon died at Napan, N. S., in 1874, aged 51 years. Mrs. Dixon died at Sackville in 1886, aged 71 years.

⁵ Amasa, only son of Edward and Eunice Lewis Dixon, married Elizabeth, daughter of Edward Bowes, Esq., late of Sackville. The children of Amasa and Elizabeth Bowes, are named Mabel Gertrude, Floyd and Edward Bowes; one other died in infancy. Mr. Dixon is a druggist and resides at Sackville, and has a prosperous business.

⁵ Eunice, eldest daughter of Edward and Eunice Lewis Dixon, married William P. Keillor, of Napan, where they reside and follow farming. They have children named Gilbert Lawrence, Hattie Maud and Emma.

⁵ Mary Emma, second daughter of Edward and Eunice Lewis Dixon, married Austin Myers, a farmer of Wentworth, N. S. Their children are Austin, Loyd, Effa and two others.

⁵ Amelia A. youngest daughter of Edward and Eunice Lewis Dixon, married George H. Longley of Waterloo, Quebec, where they resided for a time. Mrs. Longley died in 1881 aged 22 years.

⁴ Amasa, youngest son of William and Elizabeth Weldon Dixon, was also a mechanic and resided in Dorchester many years. He married Eliza Teed, daughter of Captain Mariner Teed of Westmoreland. Their children are named Albert Edward, Annie B. C. and George M. one other died in infancy. Mr. Dixon a few years since sold out his business at Dorchester and removed to Oxford N. S. where he still resides.

⁵ Albert Edward, eldest son of Amasa and Eliza Teed Dixon, married Ellen, daughter of John Smith of Sackville. He is a mechanic and resides at Dorchester.

⁵ Annie B. C. daughter of Amasa and Eliza Teed Dixon, married Thomas Brownell, carpenter. They reside at Oxford N. S.

GENEALOGY OF CHARLES DIXON, 2D.

⁵ George M. youngest son of Amasa and Eliza Teed Dixon is a carver by profession and is not married.

⁴ Elizabeth Ann, youngest daughter of William and Elizabeth Weldon Dixon, married Robert Keillor Wilbur, a farmer of Memramcook. They have children named, Jane Elizabeth Ann, Dudley Lincoln Dixon, Lytle Clarissa and Lillie May. Mr. Wilbur died in 1883. His widow still survives and resides at Dorchester.

⁵ Jane Elizabeth Ann, eldest daughter of Robert K. and Elizabeth Ann Dixon Wilbur, is married to Mr. Albert Bowser, carpenter of Dorchester, where they reside and have children named Christopher R., Robert Dudley, Nellie Blanch and one not named.

⁵ Dudley Lincoln D , son of Robert K. and Elizabeth Ann Dixon Wilbur, is a seafaring man, not married.

⁵ Lytle Clarissa, second daughter of Robert K. and Elizabeth A. Dixon Wilbur, married Hudson Grier, at present residing in California. They have no family.

⁵ Lillie May, youngest daughter of Robert K. and Elizabeth A. Dixon Wilbur, is residing in Dorchester, unmarried. Here closes the account of the family of ³ William Dixon and his wife Elizabeth Weldon.

³ Charles, second son of Charles and Rhoda Emmerson Dixon, married Jane Elisabeth Metcalf, of Point De Bute, where he settled and for a time engaged in merchandise, but subsequently turned his attention to farming. He was also a superior mechanic, an intelligent and industrious man, and a diligent reader. He died in 1867, aged 74 years. His widow survived her husband seven years. Their family bore the

names of John, Joseph, Mary, William Edwin, Charles and George E. Ritchie.

⁴ John the eldest son of Charles and Jane E. Metcalf Dixon, was also a mechanic, but gave his attention principally to farming. He married Prudence, eldest daughter of Mr. John Tingley, of Point De Bute, where they resided. Their children were named Amanda Isabel, Charles Willard, Alvin Eugene, Mary Jane, Joseph William, Victor Emanuel, Prudence Bertha and Martha Dormer. Two others died in infancy. Mr. Dixon died in 1890, aged 71 years. Mrs. Dixon still survives.

⁵ Amanda Isabel, eldest daughter of John and Prudence Tingley Dixon, married John E. Bowser, a farmer, of Sackville, where they reside. They have children, named Dixon Edward, John Willard, Jane Emmeline, Ivy Isabel and Martha Lucy.

⁵ Charles Willard, eldest son of John and Prudence Tingley Dixon, is unmarried, and spends a portion of his time on the Pacific Coast, where he has been engaged in business.

⁵ Alvin Eugene, second son of John and Prudence Tingley Dixon, married Ruth, daughter of Christopher Wry, and resides at Amherst. He is a mechanic. They have a daughter named Grace.

⁵ Mary Jane, second daughter of John and Prudence Tingley Dixon, married Mr. Amos Logan, of Amherst Point, where they follow farming. Their children are John Fremont, Mary Elizabeth, and one who died in infancy. The remaining members of the family of John and Prudence Tingley Dixon are at home, unmarried.

⁴ Joseph, second son of Charles and Jane E. Metcalf Dixon, married Martha, second daughter of John Tingley, of Point

GENEALOGY OF CHARLES DIXON, 2D. 67

De Bute. They reside at Sackville, where Mr. Dixon has been Postmaster for many years. Their children are named Minnie Jane and Arthur Wellesley.

⁵ Minnie Jane, only daughter of Joseph and Martha Tingley Dixon, married Capt. Frith Atkinson, shipmaster of Sackville, where they reside. They have no family.

⁵ Arthur Wellesley, only son of Joseph and Martha Tingley Dixon, married Elisabeth, daughter of Thomas Baird, Esq., merchant, late of Sackville. They have one child named Charles Bedford. And they keep the Intercolonial Hotel at Sackville station.

⁴ Mary, only daughter of Charles and Jane E. Metcalf Dixon, married Lemuel Bent, Esq., of Fort Lawrence. They reside at Point DeBute, and have no family, excepting an adopted daughter, named Mary, who has recently married Mr. Samuel Freeman, a wealthy farmer of Amherst, N. S.

⁴ William Edwin, third son of Charles and Jane E. Metcalf Dixon, married Augusta, daughter of Nathaniel Smith of Jollicure. They reside at Point DeBute, and follow farming. Their children are named Charity Elisabeth, and Frederic Allison.

⁵ Charity Elisabeth, only daughter of William E., and Augusta Smith Dixon, married Charles Dixon, a shipmaster, and son of Edwin Dixon, of Sackville. They had one child named Winnifred Tempest. Mr. Dixon died suddenly on shipboard about the year 1876. Mrs. Dixon and child remained at home with her parents until her recent marriage to Mr. W. B. Black, of Shimmicas, N. S.

⁵ Frederic Allison, only son of William Edwin and Augusta

Smith Dixon, married a Miss Taylor. They reside at Point De Bute, and follow farming.

⁴ Charles, fourth son of Charles and Jane E. Metcalf Dixon, died unmarried, age 22 years.

⁴ George E. Ritchie, youngest son of Charles and Jane E. Metcalf Dixon, married Miss Sarah E. Ward, of Point DeBute, where they reside. Mr. Dixon has been engaged in merchandise and farming, and is an active Justice of the Peace. The family consists of four daughters and two sons, named Amy Ella, Elmer Ellsworth, Alice Jane, Charles Leonard, Maggie May, Clara Josephine, and two others who died in infancy.

⁵ Amy Ella, eldest daughter of George E. Ritchie, and Sarah E. Ward Dixon, married H. W. Prentiss, piano maker, and resides in Boston, Mass. They have one child named Ethel.

⁵ Elmer Ellsworth, eldest son of George E. Ritchie, and Sarah E. Ward Dixon, married Miss Lucinda Ackles of Cumberland, N. S. They reside in Point DeBute, farming. They have children named Martha Jane, William Henry, and an infant. The remaining children of George E. Ritchie and Sarah E. Ward Dixon are unmarried, residing at home.

Here closes the account of the posterity of Charles Dixon and his wife Jane E. Metcalf.

³ Hannah, only daughter of Charles and Rhoda Emmerson Dixon, married Mr. John Barnes in the year 1815. They resided at Sackville. Mr. Barnes followed farming and milling until the year 1836, when he and his family, excepting the eldest daughter, removed to and settled in Wisconsin. Their family consisted of four daughters and three sons, as follows, viz: Rhoda, Rufus, Emily, Mary, John Wesley, Hannah Eliza-

beth, Charles William, and two who died in infancy. Mr. Barnes died March 25, 1854, aged 73 years, and Mrs. Barnes died July 3, 1862, aged 67 years.

⁴ Rhoda, eldest daughter of John and Hannah Dixon Barnes, married Mr. Cyrus Snell in the year 1832. Mr. Snell was engaged in milling at Sackville for a number of years. In 1853 he left Sackville and removed to Wisconsin with his family. They remained a year in Wisconsin and then removed to Spanish Fork, Utah, where they settled. Their children were named, John Wesley, George Dixon, Cryus Alma, Rufus Philips, and William Smyardus. Two others died in infancy. Mr. Snell died at Spanish Fork in 1873, aged 64 years. His death being no doubt hastened from injuries he received a short time previous, when attacked by some roughs in Salt Lake City and robbed of a considerable sum of money. Mrs. Snell still survives and continues to reside at Spanish Fork.

⁵ John Wesley, eldest son of Charles and Rhoda Barnes Snell, married Miss Anna Lucilla Beck. They reside at Spanish Fork and follow farming. Their children are Lucy Hannah, Margaret Adeline, Rhoda, Anna Lucilla, Emily Rebecca, Ellen, Joseph Herbert, Cyrus Philips, and five others who died in infancy.

⁶ Lucy Hannah, eldest daughter of John Wesley and Anna L. Beck Snell, married John W. Robertson in 1877. They reside at Spanish Fork. Their children are Ethel, Cyrus Snell, Archibald, Ralph, Bryant Barnes, Donald Whitson, Vera, and two others who died in infancy.

⁶ Margaret Adeline, second daughter of John Wesley and Anna L. Beck Snell, married James M. Creer as his second wife. They have two children, Lucilla and Sarah Jane.

⁶ Rhoda, third daughter of John Wesley and Anna L. Beck Snell, married John S. Thomas. They reside at Spanish Fork, and have children named Pratt Pace, Rhoda May, John Snell, Verna and Cyrus Grant.

⁶ Anna Lucilla, fourth daughter of John Wesley and Anna L. Beck Snell, married James M. Creer. They had one child named James Snell, who died in infancy. Mrs. Creer died June 19, 1887, aged 22 years, and Mr. Creer married her sister, as before stated.

⁶ Emily Rebecca, fifth daughter of John Wesley and Anna L. Beck Snell, married Mr. James Miller, and they have children named Elmer and Margaret.

⁵ George Dixon, second son of Cyrus and Rhoda Barnes Snell, married Sinia Dennis, of Salem, Utah. They had three children who died in childhood. Mrs. Snell died in 1868, and Mr. Snell married a second time, the name of the second wife being Miss Alexanderina McLean. They have children named Francis McLean, George Dixon, Nathan Emmerson, Alexanderina, Cyrus Edson, Irving Porter and Smyardus Philips. Mr. George D. Snell is a leading man in the community and has filled the office of Bishop of Spanish Fork since 1875 with ability and acceptance.

⁶ Francis McLean, eldest son of George Dixon and Alexanderina McLean Snell, married Miss Annie E. Thomas, of Spanish Fork, where they reside and follow milling.

The remaining children of George Dixon and Alexanderina Snell are not married.

⁵ Cyrus Alma, third son of Cyrus and Rhoda Barnes Snell, married Miss Emeline Lunceford of Callifornia, where they

GENEALOGY OF CHARLES DIXON, 2D. 71

resided. They had one daughter named Mary Rhoda. Mr. Snell died at Spanish Fork, August 5, 1863.

⁶ Mary Rhoda only daughter of Cyrus Alma and Emmeline Lunceford Snell married Mr. Charles Reed. They reside at Oakland, Cal. and have a child named Cyrus Irvin and a babe.

⁵ Rufus Philips, fourth son of Cyrus and Rhoda Barnes Snell, married Ellen Celestia Hillman, and resided at Spanish Fork. They had children named Rufus Philips, Ellen, Rhoda Emily, Adletta, John Barnes, Silas Hillman, George Alden, Heber Cyrus, William Henry, and one who died in infancy. Mrs. Snell died June 11, 1887. Mr. Rufus Philips Snell is still living at Spanish Fork with his family, who are all unmarried.

⁵ William Smyardus, youngest son of Cyrus and Rhoda Barnes Snell, died in 1889, and was never married.

⁴ Rufus, eldest son of John and Hannah Dixon Barnes, married Miss Hannah Bates. They lived in Wisconsin, and had children named Allen, George, Edwin Palmer, and Emily. At a subsequent period they removed to Iowa.

⁴ Emily, second daughter of John and Hannah Dixon Barnes married Edwin Palmer. They lived in Wisconsin, and had children named Adelaide, Edwin Franklin, John and Jennett.

⁵ Adelaide, eldest daughter of Edwin and Emily Barnes Palmer, died in childhood.

⁵ Edwin Franklin, eldest son of Edwin and Emily Barnes Palmer, was drowned when about fifteen years old.

⁵ John, the youngest son of Edwin and Emily Barnes Palmer, died August 16, 1866, at the age of 22 years.

⁵ Jennett, the youngest child of Edwin and Emily Barnes

GENEALOGY OF CHARLES DIXON, 2D.

Palmer, married James Hubbard of Milwaukee, and they have two children, one of whom is named Jennett.

Mr. Palmer died in 1864, aged 50 years, and Mrs. Palmer died in 1891.

4 Mary, third daughter of John and Hannah Dixon Barnes, married Mr. Hyrum Frank. They lived in California, and had no family. Mr. and Mrs. Frank are both dead.

4 John Wesley, second son of John and Hannah Dixon Barnes, married Miss Jennett Holmes. They reside in Wisconsin, and have children named John Fremont, Jennie M. and Frank J. The eldest of these, John Fremont, was accidentally killed at the age of twelve years.

4 Hannah Elizabeth, fourth daughter of John and Rhoda Dixon Barnes, married Mr. Henry Holmes. They reside at Dellton, Wisconsin, and have children named Herbert Lee, Frank and Lillie.

4 Charles William, youngest son of John and Hannah Dixon Barnes, is not married and resides at Dellton, Wis. He was a soldier in the Union Army, and was with General Sherman in his famed march to the Sea. Here closes the account of the posterity of Hannah Dixon and her husband, John Barnes.

3 Benjamin, youngest son of Charles and Rhoda Emmerson Dixon, married Miss Mary Weldon, daughter of Andrew Weldon, Esq., of Dorchester, about the year 1818. They resided for a time at Dorchester, and then removed to Sackville and after a few years returned to Dorchester, and from thence removed to Buctouche where they remained some ten years or upwards, and in 1845 he with his family removed to Indian Island. He was a mechanic and followed the various occupa-

GENEALOGY OF CHARLES DIXON, 2D. 73

tions of mason, miller and cooper as circumstances dictated. In early life he and his wife became members of the Methodist church, in which Mr. Dixon for many years was a zealous and effective exhorter and local preacher. His views respecting baptism having been changed, he joined the Baptist church and was employed by that body as a missionary to Charlotte County, N. B., where, as before stated, he settled his family in the year 1845. After the death of Mrs. Dixon in 1852, he married Mrs. Burnham, a widow lady residing in Lubec, Maine, and in a year or two after this marriage he went to Ohio to visit his father and family. From this visit he did not return. After visiting his relatives in Ohio he went to Michigan, and his subsequent history is unknown to his family. The family of Benjamin and Mary Weldon Dixon consisted of three sons and three daughters, as follows: James Emmerson, Rhoda Elizabeth, Ann Weldon, John W. Weldon, Esther Ann and Andrew Dale.

4 James Emmerson, eldest son of Benjamin and Mary Weldon Dixon, acquired when young an education, and followed teaching for a time. He settled at Indian Island, and married Miss Ellen Comelia Ferris in December, 1848. Their children are Richard Ferris, John Chaffy, Charles Weldon, Mary Ellen, Horace, Sidney Gordon, Arthur James and Comelia Ferris. Mrs. Dixon died March 6, 1868, aged 41 years. In 1870 Mr. Dixon married Miss Elizabeth Ferris, a sister of his first wife. No family by the second marriage. Mr. Dixon died in May 1891, aged 71 years.

5 Richard Ferris, eldest son of James E. and Ellen C. Ferris Dixon, married Miss Catharine Chaffy in 1875. They reside at

Indian Island. Their children are Halbert C., Grace E., Ethel G., Chester A., and Lottie L.

⁵ John Chaffy, second son of James E. and Ellen C. Ferris Dixon, married Miss Ada Leonard, of Leonardsville, in 1883. They reside at Indian Island, and have children named Cora L., Charles C. and Helen C.

⁵ Charles Weldon, third son of James E. and Ellen C. Ferris Dixon, married Miss Mary Chaffy of Eastport, Maine, in 1880. They reside at Indian Island, and have children named Mabel B. and Willis C.

⁵ Mary Ellen, eldest daughter of James E. and Ellen C. Ferris Dixon, married her cousin Mr. Ernest Jenks. They have no family.

⁵ Horace, the fourth son of James E. and Ellen C. Ferris Dixon, died in childhood.

⁵ Sidney Gordon, fifth son of James E. and Ellen C. Ferris Dixon, married Miss Hannah M. Cunningham, of Providence, Rhode Island, in the year 1881. Their children are named Florence E., who died in infancy, and Arthur Emmerson.

The other members of the family of James E. and Ellen C. Ferris Dixon are not married, one of whom ₅ Arthur James is a book keeper at St. John, N. B.

⁴ Rhoda Elizabeth, eldest daughter of Benjamin and Mary Weldon Dixon, was married in 1861 to Captain Frederic W. Moses, formerly of Yarmouth, England. Mr. Moses is a leading business man at Indian Island. They have no family.

⁴ Anna Weldon, second daughter of Benjamin and Mary Weldon Dixon, died in childhood.

⁴ John W. Weldon, second son of Benjamin and Mary Weldon Dixon, followed for a time the occupation of cooper,

GENEALOGY OF CHARLES DIXON, 2D.   75

with his father at Indian Island. He married in 1850, Miss Isabella Seaton French, of St. George, N. B. They removed to the United States and reside at Somerville, Mass. Their children are Benjamin Weldon, Clara B., John A., Charles Adams, Laura E, Charlotte M., and William F.

⁵ Benjamin Weldon, eldest son of John W. W., and Isabella S. French Dixon, married Miss Annie E. Irons, of Providence, in the year 1873. They reside at Brooklyn, New York, and have children named Mary Decker, Belle Seaton, Halizt Dawson, and Percy Benjamin.

⁵ Clara B., eldest daughter of John W. W., and Isabella S. French Dixon, married Henry R. Franklin of Boston, Mass, in 1874. They reside at Brooklyn, N. Y., and have children named Laura E., William Dixon and Ida Franklin.

⁵ Laura E., second daughter of John W. W., and Isabella S. French Dixon, married Edward M. Jones, of Salem, Mass., in 1882. Mrs. Jones died in the same year of her marriage.

⁵ John Adams, second son of John W. W. Dixon, resides in Maine, and is superintendent of agencies in the Mutual Life Insurance Co.

⁵ Charles Alden, third son of John W. W. and Isabella S. French Dixon, married Miss Myra Winne, of New York, in 1886, and is a partner in business with his brother Benjamin at Brooklyn.

⁵ Charlotte M., the third daughter of John W. W., and Isabella S. French Dixon, died in childhood.

⁵ William F., youngest son of John W. W. and Isabella S. French Dixon, resides at home with his parents and is not married.

⁴ Esther Ann, third daughter of Benjamin and Mary Wel-

don Dixon, married Mr. John William Jenks, at Indian Island in the year 1854. They reside at Parrsboro, N. S. Mr. Jenks is a merchant and Postmaster. Their surviving children are named Ernest Weldon, and Stuart Dixon. Three others died in childhood.

5 Ernest W. son of John W. and Esther Ann Dixon Jenks, married Miss Mary Ellen Dixon, daughter of James E. Dixon as before stated. They have no family and reside in the United States.

4 Andrew Dale, youngest son of Benjamin and Mary Weldon Dixon, resided for a time at Portland, Me., and then removed to Fall River, Mass. He married Miss Mahala Blake. Their children were named Ella and Minnie, the latter of whom is not living.

The above completes the account of the posterity of Benjamin and Mary Weldon Dixon so far as known and also the history of Charles Dixon and his wife Rhoda Emmerson and their descendants.

It will now be in order to trace out the history of Charles Dixon and Elizabeth Humphrey's family.

3 John, the eldest son of Charles and Elizabeth Humphrey Dixon, died at Miramachi when a young man and unmarried.

3 Elizabeth, eldest daughter of Charles and Elizabeth Humphrey Dixon, married Mr. John McKinlay, of Yarmouth. N. S., in the year 1824. Mr. McKinlay resided at Sackville and carried on the business of Boot and Shoe making until 1842, when he removed with his family to Ohio, and subsequently to Burlington, Iowa, where he settled and remained until his death. The family consisted of Lavina A., Jane E., John, Sarah E., Charles D., George Edward, Sidney D., Ara-

bella and one who died in infancy. Mr. McKinlay died of cholera, at Burlington in the year 1859, aged 57 years. Soon after the death of her husband Mrs. McKinlay removed with the remainder of her family to Utah and resided at Spanish Fork and at Payson. She died while visiting her daughter in Arizona in November 1890, aged 88 years nearly.

4 Lavina A., eldest daughter of John and Elizabeth Dixon McKinlay, married John M. Neely, of Burlington, Iowa, where they resided. They had one child named Cora, who with her mother died of cholera in 1851.

4 Jane E., second daughter of John and Elizabeth Dixon McKinlay, died of consumption unmarried aged 19 years.

4 John, eldest son of John and Elizabeth Dixon McKinlay, resides in California unmarried.

4 Sarah E., third daughter of John and Elizabeth Dixon McKinlay, married Enoch Reese, in the year 1850. They resided at Salt Lake City and their children are named 5 John H. and Enoch Leo. Mr. Reese died in 1876. Mrs. Reese is still living at Salt Lake City.

5 John H., eldest son of Enoch and Sarah E. McKinlay Reese, married Miss Frances E. Fox, in the year 1875. They had two children named John Roy and Enoch William, the first of whom died in infancy. Mrs. Reese died in 1888, aged 32 years. Mr. Reese, in 1890, married Miss Nora Edler, and they have one child named Sarah E. They reside in Salt Lake City. Mr. Reese is a railroad contractor.

5 Enoch Leo, youngest son of Enoch and Sarah E. McKinlay Reese, married Miss Ellen Knowlton in 1885. They have no family. Mr. Reese is engaged in the stock business and resides in Salt Lake City.

GENEALOGY OF CHARLES DIXON, 2D.

⁴ Charles D., second son of John and Elizabeth Dixon McKinlay, is not married, and resides in California.

⁴ George Edward, third son of John and Elizabeth Dixon McKinlay, resides in California. He married in 1861, Miss Caroline Springston. Their family consists of five sons and five daughters, named Sidney, Ella, George A. Eva, Ada, Lillian, Mary E., Charles, Archie and Francis, one of whom, Ella, died in childhood.

⁵ Sidney, eldest son of George and Caroline Springston McKinlay, is married and has one child.

⁴Sidney D., fourth son of John and Elizabeth Dixon McKinlay, died in 1851, of cholera, at Burlington, aged 16 years.

⁴ Arabella, youngest daughter of John and Elizabeth Dixon McKinlay, married Henry G. Boyle in the year 1865. They reside in Arizona, and have children named Henry E., Frances A., Sarah E., Charles A., Mary V., J. Reese, Heber G., Orrawell M., and one named Joseph, who died in infancy.

The account of the posterity of John and Elizabeth Dixon McKinlay, here closes.

³ Sidney, the second son of Charles and Elizabeth Humphrey Dixon, went to New Orleans about the year 1832, where he soon after died of cholera, aged 27 years. He was not married.

³ Leonard, third son of Charles and Elizabeth Humphrey Dixon, married Eliza Robson in 1832, eldest daughter of late Thomas Robson, merchant of Sackville. Leonard resided at Sackville on a portion of the property previously owned by his father, and redeemed the most of it from the wilderness. The family of Leonard and Eliza Robson Dixon consisted of four sons and one daughter, named James, Isabel, Robson

GENEALOGY OF CHARLES DIXON, 2D. 79

Morice, Henry Daniel, and Charles Thomas. Leonard Dixon was an industrious, well-meaning and highly respected man. He died in 1875, aged 67 years. Mrs. Dixon survived her husband several years.

4 James, eldest son of Leonard and Eliza Robson Dixon, when a young man about 20 years old, went to Australia. He resides at or near Ballarat, and follows mining. He is married and has children named Leonard Lincoln, Eliza, William Sherman, Isabella, Henry Francis and Charles Edmund.

4 Isabel, only daughter of Leonard and Eliza Robson Dixon, lived with her parents until they died. She was not married, and gave her attention to bringing up two orphan children of her brother's, Robson M., and Henry D. She died suddenly of paralysis in May 1887, aged fifty-two years.

4 Robson Morice, second son of Leonard and Eliza Robson Dixon, at an early age evinced a great fondness for speculation. He bought a vessel and engaged in the coasting business with some success, and then went into ship building and merchandise. He finally invested largely in an iron foundry, which did not prove a success. He married Elisabeth, youngest daughter of Christopher Boultenhouse, Esq. They had a son named Arthur Rainsford, and two other children who died in infancy. Mrs. Dixon died in 1871, aged 25 years. Robson M. Dixon died in 1874, aged 36 years.

5 Arthur Rainsford, only son of Robson M., and Elisabeth Boultenhouse Dixon is a mechanic and sometimes follows seafaring. He went to British Columbia recently. He married Lousia Deans who has a child named Hagel Elisabeth.

4 Henry Daniel, third son of Leonard and Eliza Robson Dixon, was a seafaring man and shipmaster. He married

Miss Jennie Jordan, and they had one child named Jennie Eliza. Mrs. Dixon died in 1871, and her husband Henry Dixon died in 1873, aged 33 years, leaving an orphan child.

⁵ Jennie Eliza, only child of Henry D. and Jennie Jordan Dixon, married Horatio N. Richardson, a farmer of Sackville, where they reside, and have two children, named Charles Arthur and Mabel.

⁴ Charles Thomas, youngest son of Leonard and Eliza Robson Dixon, is a farmer residing at Sackville on the homestead of his father. He married Miss Mary L. Sterling, and their children are named Eva H., James William, Charles Leonard and Thomas Henry, another died in infancy.

⁵ Eva H. only daughter of Charles Thomas and Mary L. Sterling Dixon, married Frank Phinney, Moulder of Sackville where they reside and have one child named Harold Thomas.

The other members of the family of Charles Thomas and Mary L. Sterling Dixon are not married, James William is learning telegraphy, and Charles Leonard went recently to British Columbia.

This closes the history of the family of Leonard and Eliza R. Dixon.

³ Jane, second daughter of Charles and Elizabeth Humphrey Dixon, accompanied her parents when they removed from Sackville to Kirtland, Ohio, and married George Harrison Pepper of Quincy, Illinois, in the year 1840. Their children were named Lucretia Jane, and Charles Edward. Two others died in childhood. Mr. Pepper died also at Quincy in 1852, and soon after the death of her husband, Mrs. Pepper removed from Illinois to Utah, and there was married to Wm W. Rust

in the year 1856. No children by the second marriage. Mrs. Pepper Rust died in 1879, aged 69 years.

⁴ Lucretia Jane Pepper, eldest daughter of George H. and Jane Dixon Pepper, married William C. Wightman, in the year 1855 at Salt Lake City. Their Children are named William Charles, Martha Jane, Lucretia Anna, Mary Elizabeth, Lyman Edton, Harrison Pepper. Frank Lynville, Doctor Roy, Ben Rolla and Valentine Charles. Six others died in infancy. Mr. Wightman and family reside in Payson City.

⁵ William Charles, eldest son of William C. and Lucretia J. Pepper Wightman, married Miss Harriet Sophia Jones in the year 1875 and resides at Payson City. They have children named Harriet Sophia, Laura Ethel and Cynthia Lapearl. Five others died in infancy.

⁵ Martha Jane, eldest daughter of William C. and Lucretia J. Pepper Wightman, married Horace Angolett Curtis, in the year 1875. They reside at Payson and have children named Cora Centennia, Ethel Estella, William W., Czara Allen, Martha Jane and Emma May.

⁵ Lucretia Anna, second daughter of William C. and Lucretia J. Pepper Wightman, married William Allen Miles, in the year 1882. They reside at Payson, and have children named Donna Violia, Martha Jane, Lurene and Mary Leona.

⁵ Mary Elizabeth, third daughter of William C. and Lucretia J. Pepper Wightman, married Charles Edward Vanina, of Payson. They have one child named Ruth Elda.

⁴ Charles Edward, only son of George Harrison and Jane Dixon Pepper, married Miss Adelia Webb. They have children named George Harrison, Pardon Edward, Ray and Zella. Three others died in infancy.

Here closes the account of the posterity of Jane Dixon and her husband George H. Pepper.

³ Ruth, third daughter of Charles and Elizabeth Humphrey Dixon, accompanied her parents when they removed from Sackville to Kirtland, Ohio, and in the year 1850 was married to Edward O'Hara, and resided for a time in Indiana. Mr. O'Hara's health having failed, he was advised to try a change of climate, and in 1860 went with his family to California. While there his health greatly improved and he soon after returned to Utah and settled at Payson. The children of Edward and Ruth Dixon O'Hara, are named Mary Elizabeth and Genevia and Eugenie, twins. Mr. O'Hara died in December 1886. Mrs. O'Hara still survives.

⁴ Mary Elizabeth, eldest daughter of Edward and Ruth Dixon O'Hara, married Henry Fairbanks in 1869. They reside at Payson and their children are named Henry, Edward, John B., Mary E., Charles D., Sarah V. and Mibs Morgan. One other died in childhood.

⁴ Eugenie, third daughter of Edward and Ruth Dixon O'Hara, married James Edward McCall in 1879. Their children are James Edward, Mary Eugenie, John Henry, and one other who died in infancy.

⁴ Genevia, second daughter of Edward and Ruth Dixon O'Hara, is not married and resides with her mother at Payson.

This ends the account of the posterity of Ruth Dixon and her husband Edward O'Hara.

³ Christopher Flintoff, fourth son of Charles and Elisabeth Humphrey Dixon, removed with his father's family from Sackville, N. B., to Kirtland, Ohio, in 1837. He followed farming there until the year 1861, when he with his family removed to

GENEALOGY OF CHARLES DIXON, 2D.   83

Utah and settled at Payson, where he still resides. In the year 1844 he married Miss Jane E. Wightman, of Herkimer County, New York. Their family consists of Joseph W., (who died in infancy) Ruth Elizabeth, Charles H., John Henry, Mary A., Erastus W., Emma J., Estelle V. and Christopher F. Mrs. Dixon died in 1877. Mr. Dixon still survives.

⁴ Ruth E., eldest daughter of Christopher F. and Jane E. Wightman Dixon, married David H. Kinsey in the year 1865. They resided at Salt Lake City, and had children named Stephen, David, Charles, Henrietta and Emma. Mr. Kinsey died in 1875. Mrs. Kinsey with a portion of her family still resides in the City.

⁵ David, second son of David and Ruth Elisabeth Dixon Kinsey, married Miss Martha Sargent in 1888. They reside at Provo, and had one child who died in infancy.

The other members of the family of Mr. and Mrs. Kinsey before mentioned, are not married.

⁴ Charles H., second son of Christopher F. and Jane E. Wightman Dixon, married Miss Matilda Douglass (daughter of William and Agnes Douglass) in the year 1872. Their children are named William Douglass, Charles Christopher Flintoff and Jane Elizabeth. Charles H. Dixon died at Payson in 1877, aged 29 years. His widow and children still reside at Payson.

⁴ John Henry, third son of Christopher F. and Jane E. Wightman Dixon, married Miss Eliza Jones in the year 1878. They have a daughter named Mary Jane. They reside at Payson, where Mr. Dixon is an active and leading man.

⁴ Mary A., second daughter of Christopher F. and Jane E. Wightman Dixon, married Mr. Ammon Nebekir in the year 1874. They reside at Payson and their children are named

Mary, Ann, Ammon, Aurora, Leo, Erastus, Alberta and Claudius. Of these, Mary and Erastus died in childhood.

4 Erastus W., fourth son of Christopher F. and Jane E. Wightman Dixon, resides at Payson and is not married.

4 Emma Jane, third daughter of Christopher F. and Jane E. Wightman Dixon, married Mr. Samuel Douglass in the year 1874. They reside at Payson and their children are named Mary, Armanella, Samuel, Charles, William, Emma, Henrietta Edith and Stanley.

4 Estelle V., fourth daughter of Christopher F. and Jane E. Wightman Dixon, married Joseph Fairbanks in the year 1880. They had a child named Magdalene who died in infancy.

4 Christopher F., youngest son of Christopher F. and Jane E. Wightman Dixon, married Miss Lodaska Richmond in the year 1883. They reside in Payson and have children named Cora, Emma, Marie and Christopher Flintoff.

This closes the account of the posterity of Christopher F. Dixon and his wife Jane E. Wightman.

3 Edward, fifth son of Charles and Elizabeth Humphrey Dixon, removed from Sackville, N. B. with his father's family to Ohio in 1837, where he followed farming until 1854. He crossed the Plains in company with his sisters and their families in that year and proceeded to California where he remained until 1859, when he returned to Ohio, by way of Panama and New York. He married in October 1859, Sarah Ann Gould, daughter of John Gould, Esq., of Cleveland. And in company with his brother Alfred's family in 1860 again crossed the Plains and settled in California, where he remained until 1865, when he returned to and settled at Payson, Utah, where he still resides. His family consists of three daughters and one

GENEALOGY OF CHARLES DIXON, 2D.   85

son, named Victoria Estelle, Hattie A., Ireta Elisabeth and Edward Henry. Mrs. Dixon died in the year 1882 aged 54 years. Mr. Dixon is still in good health and active.

4 Victoria Estelle, eldest daughter of Edward and Sarah A. Gould Dixon, married Edmund H. Harper, of Virginia, in the year 1879. They reside at Payson, and have children named Mabel, Ivon Dixon, Edmund H. and Sarah Ireta, the last named died in childhood.

4 Hattie A., second daughter of Edward and Sarah A. Gould Dixon, married Archibald Higham, of Salt Lake City in the year 1881. Their children are Archibald, Annie Dixon, Hattie Gould, Thomas B., and Allen Stewart. They reside at Payson.

4 Ireta Elizabeth, youngest daughter of Edward and Sarah A. Gould Dixon, married Charles W. Hemmenway, of Iowa, in the year 1885. Their children are Leigh Ireta, Charles Dixon, and Homer Gould.

4 Edward Henry, only son of Edward and Sarah A. Gould Dixon, is not married and resides at Payson with his father.

This completes the account of the posterity of Edward Dixon and his wife, Sarah A. Gould.

3 Alfred, youngest son of Charles and Elizabeth Humphrey Dixon, removed with his father, and his family, from Sackville, N. B. to Kirkland, Ohio, in 1837, where he made his home until 1843 when he went to Quincy, Ill., and studied law for a couple of years. He then went to Porter Co., Indiana, and engaged in law practice and farming, until 1860, and in April of that year he with his family, accompanied by his brother Edward and his wife, crossed the Plains with horse teams and settled in Sacramento, California. In the year 1854 he mar-

ried Miss Mary Biggart, of Ohio. Their family consisted of three sons, named George B., William E. and Charles H. Mrs. Dixon died in 1875 and in 1877 Mr. Dixon married Mrs. Julia A. Hall, of New York, a native of Sackville, N. B. About three years after this marriage, he with his wife, started to visit their native country, and in New York City Mr. Dixon was taken suddenly ill and died on the 19th of September 1880, aged 59 years.

⁴ George B., eldest son of Alfred and Mary Biggart Dixon, died in the year 1874, aged 19 years.

₄ William E., second son of Alfred and Mary Biggart Dixon, resides at Elk Grove, Sacramento Co., California, farming. He married Miss Julia I. Barnes in the year 1882. They have children named Edna Blanch, Annie Maud, Alfred Chisholm, Aubrey Ernest and Jennie Hazel.

⁴ Charles H., youngest son of Alfred and Mary Biggart Dixon, also resides at Elk Grove, California, and is engaged in farming. He married Miss Jennie L. Barnes in 1888. They have a son named George Harold.

The wives of William E. and Charles H. Dixon above mentioned, are sisters and natives of Sackville, and nieces of Mrs. Julia A. Dixon, widow of Alfred Dixon, who also resides at California. This closes the account of the posterity of Alfred Dixon and his wife Mary Biggart.

³ Mary A., fourth daughter of Charles and Elisabeth Humphrey Dixon, with her parents and their family, removed from Sackville, N. B., to Kirtland, Ohio, in 1837, and in the year 1843 she married Charles B. Wightman. They resided at Kirtland until 1862, when they removed to Utah and settled at Payson. Their children are named Amy J., Mary E.,

GENEALOGY OF CHARLES DIXON, 2D.   87

Joseph, Caroline L., Charles H., Martha E., William E., Arthur A., Abbie May, and Merton who died in infancy.

4 Amy J., oldest daughter of Charles and Mary A. Dixon Wightman, married Enoch Reese in the year 1865. They had children named Charles W., Estelle, who died at the age of 12 years, and Joseph W., one other died in infancy. Mr. Reese died in 1876. Mrs. Reese resides with her parents in Payson.

4 Mary E., second daughter of Charles B. and Mary A. Dixon Wightman, married Matthew Daly in 1863 and resides at Payson. Their children are named William C., Annie A., Matthew H., Mary J., Lillie F., Daniel P., Arthur, Graham, Caroline E., and Wilford F., another died in infancy.

4 Joseph, eldest son of Charles B. and Mary A. Dixon Wightman, married Miss Emily Johnson, in the year 1869. They reside at Payson, and have children named Joseph A., Emmeline L., Charles P., William D., Wayland R., Oran Lynn, and Dora May. Three others died in infancy.

4 Caroline L., third daughter of Charles B. and Mary Dixon Wightman, married John B. Gilbert in the year 1872. They reside at Payson, and have children named Edward F., William B., Charles, Flora, Mary A. and three who died in infancy.

4 Charles H., second son of Charles B. and Mary Dixon Wightman, married Lavinia Collett, in 1873, and resides in Payson. Their children are Myrtle, Effie, Frank, Caroline, Martha, William, and one who died in infancy.

4 Martha E., fourth daughter of Charles B. and Mary Dixon Wightman, married C. W. Morrill in 1873. They reside in Montana. They have children named Martha A., Madora, Lillie Pearl, Mary Hannah and Charles Joseph.

4 William E., third son of Charles B. and Mary Dixon

Wightman, married Miss Effie Wyman in Butte City, Montana, where they reside. They have no family.

⁴ Arthur A. and ⁴ Abbie May, children of Charles B. and Mary Dixon Wightman, are not married.

The account of the posterity of Mary Dixon and her husband Charles B. Wightman is here closed.

³ Martha, youngest daughter of Charles and Elisabeth Humphrey Dixon, with her parents and their family, removed from Sackville, N. B., to Kirtland, Ohio, in 1837. She became a member of the Church of Latter Day Saints soon after her arrival at Kirtland, and has remained to the present a zealous and consistent member thereof. In the year 1846 she married Mr. Orrawell Simons, of New Hampshire, at Kirtland, where they resided until April, 1854, when they, with her brother Edward, started upon their journey across the Plains to Utah, arriving at Salt Sake City in September. From there they proceeded to Spanish Fork, where they spent the winter in a Fort built to protect them from the Indians. In the spring of 1855 they removed to Payson and settled, where they still reside. In 1876 Mr. and Mrs. Simons visited the Centennial at Philadelphia, and from thence proceeded to Sackville, visiting their relatives and friends in that vicinity, and then returned to Utah. The family of Orrawell and Martha Dixon Simons consists of Elizabeth A., Edward, Orrawell, Martha, Albert Lee, Enos Wells, Major Gustavus and two others who died in infancy.

⁴ Elizabeth A., eldest daughter of Orrawell and Martha Dixon Simons, married Thomas G. Wimmer, of Iowa, in 1866. They reside at Payson and have children named Thomas G., Emily E., Robert S., Martha L., Ethel G., William L., Susan

GENEALOGY OF CHARLES DIXON, 2D.   89

Lyle, Leland Wayne, Hazel and a babe. Three others died in childhood.

5 Thomas G., eldest son of Thomas G. and Elizabeth A. Simons Wimmer, married Sarah E. Patten in 1886. They reside at Payson, and have two sons named Lloyd P. and Andy G.

5 Emily E., eldest daughter of Thomas G. and Elizabeth A. Simons Wimmer, married Andrew J. Shore in the year 1889. Mr. Shore is a medical doctor residing at Payson. They have one child named Rexford.

4 Edward, eldest son of Orrawell and Martha Dixon Simons, married Miss Julia Collett in the year 1874. They reside at Payson, and have children named Orrawell, Pearl, Delpha, Lynn and Ruby, another died in infancy.

4 Orrawell, second son of Orrawell and Martha Dixon Simons, married Miss Frances M. Brewerton in 1884. They reside at Payson, and have children named Rhea, Major O. and Martha B.

4 Martha second daughter of Orrawell and Martha Dixon Simons, married Lyman Kapple in 1881. They reside at Payson, and have children named Lyman, Albert S. and Orrawell. One other died in infancy

4 Albert Lee, third son of Orrawell and Martha Dixon Simons, married Miss Elizabeth Knights. They have children named Ethel, Albert Lee and Leland K.

4 Enos Wells, fourth son of Orrawell and Martha Dixon Simons, married Miss Elizabeth R. Pickering in 1886. They reside at Payson and have children named Donna and Enos Wells.

[4] Major Gustavus, youngest son of Orrawell and Martha Dixon Simons, died in 1878 in the eleventh year of his age.

The account of the posterity of Martha Dixon and her husband Orrawell Simons here closes.

The foregoing comprises the historical and genealogical record of the posterity of Charles Dixon the second by his wives Rhoda Emmerson and Elizabeth Humphrey.

Posterity of Charles Dixon, second:

	Born.	Living.	Dead.
Children	16	5	11
Grand "	85	56	29
Great Grand "	283	225	58
Great Great Grand "	137	117	20
Great Great Great Grand "	21	18	3
	542	421	121

GENEALOGY OF SUSANNAH DIXON AND HER HUSBAND GEORGE BULMER.

CHAPTER IV.

²SUSANNAH DIXON, the second daughter of Charles and Susannah Coates Dixon, married George Bulmer, in the year 1784. Mr. Bulmer, as previously stated, came when a lad of 12 years of age from England in the same ship with Mr. Dixon and his family, and a few years subsequently, his mother and several of her sons came out and settled near Amherst, where some of their descendants still remain. The Bulmer family is said to be of Norman descent. Mr. George Bulmer purchased a large lot of land adjoining the farm of his father-in-law, which he industriously improved and cultivated for many years, until he became somewhat deranged, and this affliction having assumed a somewhat alarming aspect it was deemed necessary in the interests of his family to invoke the action of the Court of Chancery; and a decree was obtained by which the property was placed in the hands of Commissioners, who should control the same for the maintenance of Mr. and Mrs. Bulmer and in the interest of the family. Mr. and Mrs. Bulmer both survived for many years after the above action was taken. Mrs. Bulmer died in 1835 aged 67 years, and Mr. Bulmer in 1841 aged 82 years.

The author has not been able to obtain access to the family register of George and Susanna Dixon Bulmer, or to any data showing the exact date of their marriage or the births of their children, but from the circumstances that have come to his knowledge he believes the following to be correct:

Jane, born in 1785. Charles, born in 1787.
James B., born in 1789. Mary, born in 1791.
John, born in 1793. George, born in 1795.
Ann, born in 1797. Elizabeth, born in 1799.
Isabel, born in 1801. Edward, born in 1803.
H. Nelson, born in 1807. William, born in 1809.
Ruth, born in 1811.

3 Jane, the eldest daughter of George and Susanna Dixon Bulmer, married William Smith, a farmer. This marriage took place about 1805. They settled at Maccan, N. S. Mr. Smith was a local preacher among the Methodists. He was a very large, robust person, and owing to some accident he was obliged to have one of his limbs amputated just below the knee, and the author remembers seeing him wearing an immense wooden leg. The family of William Smith and Jane Bulmer were named Elizabeth, George, Henry, Susan, Ann, Mary and John Nelson. Mrs. Smith died about the year 1830. Mr. Smith married a Miss Harrison, and the time of his death is unknown. He had some family by his second wife.

4 Elisabeth, eldest daughter of William and Jane Bulmer Smith, married Samuel Horton about the year 1834. Mr. Horton was a mechanic, a diligent industrious man, a native of Sackville, where he resided until the end of iife. They both became members of the Methodist church in 1836 and remained to the end in that connection. They had children named

AND HER HUSBAND, GEORGE BULMER.

Henry, Elizabeth, Amanda, Charlotte and George, all of whom except the last named died unmarried of consumption. Mr. Horton died in 1873 aged 68 years, and Mrs. Horton died in 1882, aged 77.

5 George, the youngest son of Samuel and Elizabeth Smith Horton, married Annie Crossman, daughter of Mr. Samuel Crossman of Fairfield. They resided at Fairfield and had children named Emma and Annie May. Mr. Horton died of consumption also in the year 1879 aged 30.

4 George, eldest son of William and Jane Bulmer Smith, married Esther Brown of Maccan, where they resided. They had children named Jerusha Jane, John W., Thomas B., Tillott H. and Stephen M.

5 Jerusha Jane, eldest daughter of George and Esther Brown Smith, married Thomas Boss in 1854. They reside at Spring Hill and have children named Cynthia Selina, Burton, Sarah Esther, Moses Yonng, Azeal Wellington, Rupert Cellar and one died in infancy.

6 Cynthia Selina Boss, eldest daughter of Thomas and Jerusha Jane Smith Boss is married.

6 Burton Boss, eldest son of Thomas and Jernsha Jane Smith Boss, is married and has children named William Farmer, Lillie May, Janet Murella and Della Lavinia.

6 Sarah Esther Boss, second daughter of Thomas and Jerusha Jane Smith Boss, married a Mr. McAloney and they have one child named Thomas William. The remaining members of Thomas and Jerusha Jane Smith Boss' family are not married.

5 John W., 5 Thomas B. and 5 Tillott H., sons of George and Esther Brown Smith, are married and the first named has

seven children and the others two children each, and one grand child each.

⁴ Susan, second daughter of William and Jane Bulmer Smith, married Andrew Herrett. They had children named Augusta, Jane, Phoebe, Mary, David, Ambrose and Eliza, all of whom except Phoebe and Eliza are married and have families, as follows: ₅ Augusta has six children, ⁵ Jane has seven, ⁵ Mary has four,⁵ David has eight and ⁵ Ambrose has five children.

⁴ Ann, third daughter of William and Jane Bulmer Smith, married John Atkinson in the year 1846. They resided at Maccan, N. S., and followed farming. Their children are Thomas Henry, William Smith, Eunice Ann and Ella Jane. Mrs. Atkinson died in 1877 and Mr. Atkinson still survives.

⁵ Thomas Henry, the eldest son of John and Ann Smith Atkinson, was drowned when about 10 years of age.

⁵ William Smith, second son of John and Ann Smith Atkinson, married Cecilia Quinn in 1872, and had children named Eva Grace, Henry Allison and Ella Jane.

⁵ Eunice Ann, eldest daughter of John and Ann Smith Atkinson, married George K. Nullall in 1874, and they have children named Timothy Egbert, Moulton and George.

⁵ Ella Jane, youngest daughter of John and Ann Smith Atkinson, married Thomas Stewart in 1877. They had children named Laura May, Moreton and Irene. Mrs. Stewart died in 1885, and shortly after her death Mr. Stewart and the eldest daughter died.

⁴ Mary, fourth daughter of William and Jane Bulmer Smith, married Nathan Boss in 1841. They have family named Sarah Elizabeth, Ruth, Augusta, Susan Jane, Henry Smith and James Tweedy, who are, most of them married

and have families, said to number twelve children and several grand children.

[4] John N., youngest son of William and Jane Bulmer Smith, married Elizabeth Harrison about the year 1846. They have children named William A., Alice A., Caroline A., Thomas H., Adelaide B., Charles A., James E., Leonard J., Walter R. and Harvey N. Of the above named,[5] William A. is married and has three children, [5] Alice A. is married and has seven children, [5] Carolin A. is married and has seven children, [5] Thomas H. is married and has three children, and [5] James E. is married and has two children.

The foregoing comprises all the information the writer was able to obtain relating to the posterity of Jane Bulmer and her husband, William Smith, and its imperfection and incompleteness is much regretted.

[3] Charles D., eldest son of George and Susanna Dixon Bulmer, married Elizabeth Oulton of Westmoreland, in the year 1809. They settled at Sackville upon a piece of land which his grandfather, Charles Dixon, gave him as his namesake. Mr. Bulmer was an industrious and enterprising man and soon turned the wilderness into fruitful fields. He was not only a good farmer, but he turned his attention after a time to lumbering and milling with some success. Their family consisted of Jane Oulton, Charles Dixon, George Nelson, Rufus Smith, Matilda, Charity, Edwin Oulton, Abigail and William Crane. Mr. Bulmer died in 1864, aged 77 years, and his wife died in 1870, aged 83 years.

[4] Jane O., eldest daughter of Charles D. and Elizabeth Oulton Bulmer, married Titus Anderson, son of Thomas Anderson, of Cole's Island, in 1830. Titus Anderson became

a seafaring man shortly after his marriage, and in a little time a ship master in the coasting trade, an occupation he followed the greater part of his life, and in which he unfortunately lost his life. The vessel he commanded being wrecked by being driven ashore at St. John Cape, when he and a young lad were drowned. This event occurred the 8th of July, 1870. Mr. Anderson was about 60 years of age. His widow is still living and residing in Sackville, N. B. Their family consisted of George, Ammi, Charles Marshall, Thomas Reece, Gaius, and an adopted daughter named Sarah.

[5] George, eldest son of Titus and Jane O. Bulmer Anderson married Arabella Ayr, son of Jesse Ayr. They resided at Sackville, and their family consisted of Rupert T., Ernest L., Jesse E., Carrie Bell and one who died in infancy. Mr. Anderson, or as he was generally called Captain George, early in life became engaged in the sea-faring and coasting business which he followed with success. He then became engaged in shipbuilding in company with his brother Ammi, which he followed for a few years. His death occurred in March 1872. Mrs. Anderson died in March 1879.

[6] Rupert T., eldest son of George and Arabella Ayr Anderson, is a shipmaster and not married.

[6] Ernest L. second son of George and Arabella Ayr Anderson is also a shipmaster and is married to Miss Jessie Ford, daughter of Mr. Alexander Ford, of Moncton, N. B.

[5] Jesse Edwin, youngest son of George and Arabella Ayr Anderson, is also a seafaring man and is not married.

[6] Carrie Bell, only daughter of George and Arabella Ayr Anderson, is not married.

[5] Ammi, second son of Titus and Jane O. Bulmer Ander-

son, was an excellent mechanic, and followed his occupation pretty closely for many years. He was also at one time engaged in shipbuilding and ship owning with his brother George as previously stated. He married Elizabeth, eldest daughter of Charles D. Bulmer, and their family consisted of two children both of whom died in childhood. Mr. Anderson died very suddenly in February 1885, aged 52. His widow survived until February 1891 when she also died.

5 Charles Marshall, third son of Titus and Jane O. Bulmer Anderson, also became a seafaring man and shipmaster which he successfully followed for a number of years. He first married Mary E. Wry, daughter of Isaac Wry, of Sackville. She died in 1878, leaving her husband with a little daughter named Mary E. One other died in infancy. Mr. Anderson married again in 1873, Miss Bertha Dixon, daughter of John W. Dixon, of Dorchester, N. B., where he resided for a time and subsequently removed to New Zealand, as stated in a previous chapter.

5 Thomas Reese, fourth son of Titus and Jane O. Bulmer Anderson, is also a shipmaster and stands high in his profession. He married Miss Ruth Eliza Cole, who accompanied her husband on a sea voyage and died on shipboard in November, 1864. Captain Thomas has not married a second time, and resides at Sackville with his mother when not absent on sea voyages.

5 Gaius youngest son of Titus and Jane O. Bulmer Anderson, married Emma A., daughter of Robert Keillor, Esq., of Amherst, N. S., in 1865, and shortly afterwards removed to Fiji, where they still reside, engaged in agricultural pursuits.

They have children named Emma Ruth, Lucy Ann, Robert Gaius and Minnie Alice.

⁴ Charles D., eldest son of Charles D., and Elizabeth Oulton Bulmer, married Jane Carter, daughter of Thomas Carter of Dorchester. Mr. Bulmer in early life followed seafaring, and after his marriage he was engaged in lumbering, milling and other pursuits. They resided at Sackville, and had a family named Elizabeth, Charles, Lucinda, Ezra, Albert, William, Amos, Jane and Linda twins, and Rufus and one died in childhood. Mr. Bulmer died in 1876, aged 6¼ years. Mrs. Bulmer still survives.

⁵ Elizabeth, eldest daughter of Charles D. and Jane Carter Bulmer, married Ammi Anderson as before stated.

⁵ Charles, eldest son of Charles D. and Jane Carter Bulmer, when quite young went to California. When last heard from he was in the lumber business and not married.

⁵ Lucinda, second daughter of Charles D. and Jane Carter Bulmer, married a Mr. Scott, of Nova Scotia. They had one child named Albert. Mrs. Scott subsequently became deranged and is now an inmate of the Provincial Lunatic' Asylum, and her child found a home with Mrs. Ammi Anderson.

⁵ Ezra, second son of Charles D. and Jane Carter Bulmer, died unmarried, aged 25 years.

⁵ Albert, third son of Charles D. and Jane Carter Bulmer, was a seafaring man, and when last heard from was at Greenock, Scotland, and not married.

⁵ William, fourth son of Charles D. and Jane Carter Bulmer, died in 1865, aged 17 years.

⁵ Amos, fifth son of Charles D. and Jane Carter Bulmer, is a mechanic and resides at Sackville. He married Julia, daugh-

ter of Isaac B. Baines. They have children, named Blanche, John and Amos Seymour.

⁵ Jane, third daughter of Charles D. and Jane Carter Bulmer, married William Jones, of Point de Bute, but died shortly after her marriage, in the year 1886, leaving no child.

⁵ Linda, youngest daughter of Charles D. and Jane Carter Bulmer, married William King, farmer, of Woodville, about 1889.

⁵ Rufus, youngest son of Charles D. and Jane Carter Bulmer, married Miss Griselda McDonald, of Bathurst, N. B. He is an engine driver and resides at Moncton. They have children, named Janey, Bessie and Thomas.

⁴ George Nelson, second son of Charles D. and Elizabeth Oulton Bulmer, married Lavinia, daughter of Nathan Merrill, in 1840. They settled at Sackville, on the farm formerly owned by John Barnes and also by Cyrus Snell. Mr. Bulmer followed milling with fair success. The family consisted of Alma, Bedford, Melissa, Richard, Seth and Emma Alice; two others died in childhood. Mrs. Bulmer died in October, 1877, and her husband in December, 1890.

⁵ Alma, the eldest child of George N. and Lavinia Merrill Bulmer, died in 1864, unmarried, aged 24 years.

⁵ Bedford, second child of George N. and Lavinia Merrill Bulmer, married Sarah Anderson, adopted daughter of Titus Anderson, and resides in New Zealand and is engaged in farming and lumbering. They have children, named Auta Alice, Florence, Frank, Arthur, George and Philip.

⁵ Melissa, third child of George N. and Lavinia Merrill Bulmer, married Mr. Frederick Hunter, a machinist, residing at Moncton.

⁵ Richard, fourth child of George N. and Lavinia Merrill Bulmer, married Miss Jane Anderson. They reside at Virginia City, Nevada, where they are engaged in mining and other pursuits. They have children, named Frederic Bruce, Roscoe Bayard, George and Halbert.

⁵ Seth, fifth child of George N. and Lavinia Merrill Bulmer, married Elvira, daughter of H. Nelson Bulmer, of Sackville. They reside on the property occupied recently by the said George N. Bulmer, and follow milling, lumbering and farming. They have no children.

⁵ Emma Alice, youngest child of George N. and Lavinia Merrill Bulmer, married Daniel McQuarrie, engine driver, of Moncton, where they reside.

⁴ Rufus Smith, third son of Charles D. and Elizabeth Oulton Bulmer, is a farmer, residing upon the homestead of his late father. In 1846 he married Ruth Merrill, a daughter of Nathan Merrill, and their children are named Jane Elizabeth, Annie Laura, Sarah Alice, Nathan H. and Addie V. A few years subsequent to his marriage Mr. Bulmer had the misfortune to have one of his legs very badly fractured, and after recovery had it again accidentally broken, and when, after a long time he finally recovered, the limb was found to be some inches shorter than the other, rendering him quite lame. Mrs. Bulmer died in July, 1886. Mr. Bulmer survives.

⁵ Jane Elizabeth, eldest daughter of Rufus Smith and Ruth Merrill Bulmer, married John Estabrooks, a carpenter, of Sackville, who had before been married to Mary Ann, daughter of James B. Bulmer. The children of the second marriage are Lena Ruth, Queen and another.

AND HER HUSBAND, GEORGE BULMER.

⁵ Annie Laura, second daughter of Rufus S. and Ruth Merrill Bulmer, is not married and resides at home.

⁵ Sarah Alice, third daughter of Rufus S. and Ruth Merrill Bulmer, married James Turner Bulmer, son of William C. Bulmer, of Sackville, where they reside, and follow farming. They have no family.

⁵ Nathan H., only son of Rufus S. and Ruth Merrill Bulmer, is a farmer, residing upon the farm of his father. He married Minnie, only daughter of William C. Bulmer, above named. Their children are Laura Tynon and Henry Irving.

⁵ Addie V., youngest daughter of Rufus S. and Ruth Merrill Bulmer, married Mr. Adam Carter, of Westmoreland, where they reside and follow farming. Their children are James Emery, Garth Merrill and another not named.

⁴ Matilda, second daughter of Charles D. and Elizabeth Oulton Bulmer, died unmarried, having perished in the flames when her father's house was burned in the year 1849.

⁴ Charity, the third daughter of Charles D. and Elizabeth Oulton Bulmer, married William Teed, of Westmoreland. He was a seafaring man. They had one daughter, named Ann. Mr. Teed died of consumption within a short period, and Mrs. Teed subsequently married Capt. Thomas Lowerison, of Westmoreland, and there resided until her death in 1878, in the 56th year of his age. The family of Thomas Lowerison and Charity Bulmer Teed consists of Jane, Isabel, Fanny, Emma Ruth, Melissa, Robert O., Zerbinett, and three others who died in infancy.

⁵ Anne Teed, only daughter of William and Charity Bulmer Teed, married James S. Lowerison, of Westmoreland.

They have children, named William and Roy and a daughter who died in childhood.

⁵ Jane, eldest daughter of Thomas and Charity B. Teed Lowerison, married Clarence Brownell, a farmer, residing at Amherst. They have children, named Ellsworth, Avess, Fanny, Belle and another.

⁵ Isabel, second daughter of Thomas and Charity B. Teed Lowerison, is a dress-maker, residing at Sackville, and not married.

⁵ Fanny, third daughter of Thomas and Charity B. Teed Lowerison, married John Cove, a mechanic, residing at Sackville. They have children, named Ivy and Weeny Belle.

⁵ Emma Ruth, fourth daughter of Thomas and Charity B. Teed Lowerison, married David Carter, section foreman on the I. C. Railway.

⁵ Melissa, fifth daughter of Thomas and Charity B. Teed Lowerison, married Charles Brown, son of Daniel Brown, of Tongue's Island, where they reside. The remaining surviving children of Thomas and Charity B. Teed Lowerison are not married.

⁴ Edwin O., fourth son of Charles D. and Elizabeth Oulton Bulmer, married Eliza Teed, who died of consumption within two years, leaving an infant child, which also died in a short time. He then married Charity Ogden, and their family consists of Ammi, Bamford, Sidney, Rachael, Elizabeth Lawson, Clara, Julia, Dora May, Effa and George M.; three others died in infancy. They resided at Sackville for a time and then removed to or near Woodstock, Carleton county, N. B., where they still remain and are farming.

⁵ Ammi, the eldest son of Edwin O. and Charity Ogden Bul-

mer, married Elizabeth Haywood, of Carleton, and they reside at Northampton, and have children named Lena, Frank and another.

5 Bamford, second son of Edwin O. and Charity Ogden Bulmer, married Mary Wry, widow of John Wry. They reside at Northampton, farming, and their children are named Emma, Milly, Harmon, Clarence, Charles, and one not named.

5 Rachel, eldest daughter of Edwin O. and Charity Ogden Bulmer, married Alfred Murphy. They have one child.

5 Clara, third daughter of Edwin O. and Charity Ogden Bulmer, is married and resides at Woodstock.

5 Julia, fourth daughter of Edwin O. and Charity Ogden Bulmer, died in 1887, aged 23 years. The remaining children of Edwin O. and Charity Ogden Bulmer are unmarried.

4 Abigail, youngest daughter of Charles D. and Elizabeth Oulton Bulmer, married John Mayberry, a mechanic. They resided at Haverhill, Mass. They had one daughter, who is married to Henry Felch, and they reside at Ashland, New Hampshire, and have no family. Mr. Mayberry died about the year 1880, and Mrs. Mayberry is still living, residing with her daughter at Ashland.

4 William Crane, youngest son of Charles D. and Elizabeth Oulton Bulmer, married Sarah Ann, daughter of H. Nelson Bulmer. He is a machinist, and resides at Moncton, and is employed in the Government Railway Works there. Their family consists of Harold, Florence and Charles. Milly Louise and Eliza died, one at 14 and the other at 17 years of age, and four others died in childhood.

5 Harold, the eldest son of William C. and Sarah Ann Bulmer, is also a machinist and employed in the Government

works at Moncton, and is not married. The remaining members of the family of William C. and Sarah Ann Bulmer are unmarried and at home with their parents. This closes the account of the family of Charles D. Bulmer and his wife, Elizabeth Oulton.

3 James B., second son of George and Susannah Dixon Bulmer, married Ruth Harris, eldest daughter of John Harris and grand-daughter of William Cornforth, one of the early settlers of Sackville. Mr. and Mrs. Bulmer settled at Sackville on land which formed a part of the Cornforth Estate and followed farming. They had children named William Cornforth, Rebecca, Edward, Susan, George, Mary Ann, John and Hazen B.; one other died in childhood. Mr. Bulmer died in 1842, aged 63 years. Mrs. Bulmer died in 1874, aged 78 years. They were both members of the Methodist Church.

4 William C., eldest son of James B. and Ruth Harris Bulmer, married Jane, daughter of Joseph Richardson, and settled on a piece of new and unimproved land which formed a portion of the Bulmer estate. With great industry and carefulness they redeemed the land from the wilderness and converted it into fruitful fields and surrounded themselves with evidences of prosperity. They had children named Joseph Benson, Frank James Turner and Minnie and five others who died in infancy. Mrs. Bulmer died in 1889, aged 68 years. Mr. Bulmer survives.

5 Joseph B., eldest son of William C. and Jane Richardson Bulmer, married Martha, daughter of Chipman Chase, of Woodpoint, N. B. They reside at Sackville on a part of the Bulmer property and are engaged in farming. They have no children.

5 Frank, second son of William C. and Jane Richardson Bulmer, is married to Miss Martha O'Neil, of Moncton.

5 James Turner, youngest son of William C. and Jane Richardson Bulmer, resides on the homestead of his father, farming, and is married to Sarah Alice, daughter of Rufus S. Bulmer, as stated on page 101.

5 Minnie, only daughter of William C. and Jane Richardson Bulmer, married Nathan H., only son of Rufus S. Bulmer, as stated page 101.

4 Rebecca, eldest daughter of James B. and Ruth Harris Bulmer, went to the United States, where she married Mr. James Tynon. They subsequently settled at Denver, Colorado, where they still reside, and have one daughter named Adeline, who is not married and resides with her parents.

4 Edward, second son of James B. and Ruth Harris Bulmer, was an excellent mechanic. He settled at Sackville and married Sophia Blanch, who died in a brief period after her marriage. Mr. Bulmer subsequently married Lydia Briggs. They had one son named Frederic. Mr. Bulmer died in July 1864, aged 48 years. His widow is married again to James Wry.

5 Frederic, only child of Edward and Lydia Briggs Bulmer, married a Miss Tower of Rockport, and resides in Massachusetts, and has one son.

4 Susan, second daughter of James B. and Ruth Harris Bulmer, married George Bowser of Sackville, as his second wife. They had no family, and Mrs. Bowser died in 1886, aged 58 years.

4 George, third son of James B. and Ruth Harris Bulmer, is also an excellent mechanic, and resides at Westmoreland.

He married Miss Fanny Fowler, daughter of the late Amos Fowler of Westmoreland. Their family consists of Walter, James, Charles, and Arthur, and two others who died in childhood. Mr. Bulmer, some years ago visited his sister at Denver, Colorado, and finding remunerative employment there prolonged his visit for a considerable time, and shortly after his return home, Mrs. Bulmer being on a visit to St. John for a few days was was taken ill and died very suddenly in the year 1889. None of the children of George and Fanny Fowler Bulmer are married.

4 Mary Ann, third daughter of James B. and Ruth Harris Bulmer, married Mr. John Estabrooks, a mechanic of Sackville, where they resided. They had children named Annie and Maggie. Mrs. Estabrooks died in 1865, aged 30 thirty years. Mr. Estabrooks subsequently married Jane Elizabeth, daughter of Rufus S. Bulmer, as stated on page 100.

4 John, fourth son of James B. and Ruth Harris Bulmer, was a blacksmith, and went to Boston, where he resided until his death, which occured in 1882, at the age of forty-five years. He was married in the United States but had no family.

4 Hazen B., youngest son of James B. and Ruth Harris Bulmer, is also a mechanic, and unmarried, residing at Sackville. This closes the account of James B. and Ruth Harris Bulmer.

3 Mary, second daughter of George and Susannah Dixon Bulmer, married Benjamin C. Scurr, a farmer and also a mechanic. Benjamin Scurr was the only child of Thomas Scurr and Elizabeth Cornforth, who were married in August, 1787. Benjamin C. Scurr was born June 30, 1788. His mother died within a week after his birth, and the infant was placed in the

care of Mrs. Jonathan Burnham, (his mother's sister), where he remained until he became a man. His father, Thomas Scurr, soon after the death of his wife sailed on a voyage to the West Indies, and never having returned, is supposed to have been lost at sea. Benjamin C. Scurr settled upon a piece of new and unimproved land in Sackville, and by industry and perseverance soon brought it under good cultivation and became a prosperous and successful farmer. The children of Benjamin C. and Mary Bulmer Scurr were Elizabeth Ann, Susan, Ruth Grace, Charles and Thomas. Mr. Scurr died in 1853, aged 64 years, and Mrs. Scurr died in 1866, aged 75 years.

4 Elizabeth Ann, eldest daughter of Benjamin C. and Mary Bulmer Scurr, married Jonathan C. Black, eldest son of Samuel Black of Halifax, N. S. They resided at Sackville. Mr. Black enaged for a time in merchandise, and also in farming, and for several years filled the position of Deputy Treasurer and Comptroller of Customs. Their family consists of four sons and three daughters, named Samuel, Mary, Albert, Rebecca, Benjamin Scurr, Louisa and William. Mr. Black died in 1857, aged 43 years. His widow subsequently married James Ayr as his second wife. Mrs. Ayr. died in 1865, aged 51 years.

5 Samuel, eldest son of Jonathan C. and Elizabeth Ann Scurr Black, married Mary, daughter of Reuben Watts. They removed to Calais, Me., where they still reside. Their children are named Howard, Florence, Frank and Charles Albert.

6 Florence, only daughter of Samuel Black, married a Mr. Read of Boston. They reside in Massachusetts and have one child.

5 Mary, the eldest daughter of Jonathan C. and Elizabeth

Ann Scurr Black, married William Boultenhouse, son of the late Christopher Boultenhouse, shipbuilder of Sackville. They resided at Sackville and had two daughters, named Minnie and Rebecca. Mr. Boultenhouse died in 1860, aged 38 years. Mrs. Boultenhouse removed with her daughters to Philadelphia where they still reside.

5 Albert, second son of Jonathan C. and Elizabeth Ann Scurr Black, married Rebecca Teed, of Sackville. He is an excellent mechanic. He resided at Sackville for many years, but recently removed to or near Boston. Their children are Alexander, Mary, Carrie, Benjamin S. and Charles Albert. Four others died in childhood.

5 Rebecca, second daughter of Jonathan C. and Elizabeth Ann Scurr Black married George T. Bowser, a retired farmer, of Sackville. They have no family.

5 Benjamin Scurr, third son of Jonathan C. and Elizabeth Ann Scurr Black, married a Miss Marshall, of St. John, where they reside, and Mr. Black occupies a prominent position in the office of the Western Union Telegraph Company. They have no family.

5 Louise, youngest daughter of Jonathan C. and Elizabeth Ann Scurr Black, married John T. Carter, son of the late Thomas Carter, of Sackville, where they reside and follow farming. Their children are named Cora, Thomas and Hattie.

6 Cora, eldest daughter of John T. and Louise Black Carter, married Charles Weldon in 1889. Mr. Weldon is a son of Mr. Ovid Weldon, of Sackville, where they reside and follow farming.

6 Thomas, only son of John T. and Louise Black Carter, went to British Columbia in 1890, and was employed on board

AND HER HUSBAND, GEORGE BULMER. 109

a steamer, from which he, with another young man from Sackville named Purdy, accidentally fell overboard and were lost. This event occurred in the 21st year of his age.

5 William, the youngest son of Jonathan C. and Elizabeth Ann Scurr Black, is married and resides in Pennsylvania, and has children named Ella May, Ida Louise, Rebecca Victoria and Clarence William.

4 Susan, second daughter of Benjamin C. and Mary Bulmer Scurr, married Mr. Solomon Killam, Leather manufacturer, in 1836. Mr. Killam died in 1837. After Mr. Killam's death, the widow returned to her father's house, where she remained until 1842, when she married James Smith, a prosperous farmer residing at Fort Lawrence. Their family consisted of three sons and one daughter named Isabel Ruth, Charles Albert, Martin and Benjamin Scurr. Mr. Smith died in 1868. His widow still survives.

5 Isabel Ruth, eldest daughter of James and Susan Scurr Smith, married Shelby H. Kifer, a farmer. They reside in California and have a family, named Susie, Isabel, Flora, Lillie, Annie Louise and Shelby. One other died in infancy.

5 Charles Albert, eldest son of James and Susan Scurr Smith, married Eliza Mills, and resides at Fort Lawrence farming. Mr. Smith is a very ingenious man, and has constructed machinery of various kinds, and is engaged in manufacturing lumber by machinery of his own construction. The family of Charles Albert and Eliza Mills Smith consists of Alice, James Edgar, Moreley, Joseph, Nora, Ann, Emma, Julia, Mabel and Blanche, all at home and unmarried except 6 Alice who has just been married to John Carter, son of Joseph Carter, of Point de Bute.

⁵ Martin, second son of James and Susan Scurr Smith, married Louisa Lawrence, daughter of Gilbert Lawrence, Esq., He resides at Fort Lawrence upon the homestead of his father. His children are named Belle, Fred, Edith, Jennie Louise, ~~Louise~~, Elvie and David Walter.

⁶ Belle, the eldest daughter of Martin and Louisa Lawrence Smith, is married to William, eldest son of Albert Fawcett of Sackville, where they reside and follow farming. They have one child. The remaining members of the family of Martin and Louisa Lawrence Smith are not married.

⁵ Benjamin Scurr, youngest son of James and Susan Scurr Smith, died in 1883, unmarried. He was induced to attend a Charivari party at Mount Whately, at which he was shot and almost instantly killed. Whether the sad result was accidental or otherwise has never been satisfactorily ascertained.

⁴ Ruth Grace, youngest daughter of Benjamin C. and Mary Bulmer Scurr, married Jesse L. Bent, in October 1839. Jesse was the only son of Vose Bent, of Fort Lawrence. They resided at Fort Lawrence for some years, and afterward removed to Sackville, and Mr. Bent engaged in merchandise. He was for many years a leading magistrate, and transacted a large amount of business in that capacity. They had no family. Mrs. Bent died in 1886, aged 68. Mr. Bent died in 1889.

⁴ Charles, eldest son of Benjamin C. and Mary Bulmer Scurr, resides at Sackville, on a portion of what was his Father's farm, and is an industrious and successful farmer. He married Eunice, youngest daughter of John Patterson, of Cole's Island. Their children are Benjamin, John and Annie; and one died in infancy.

⁵ Benjamin, eldest son of Charles and Eunice Patterson

AND HER HUSBAND, GEORGE BULMER.

Scur, married Miss Georgiana Ayr, daughter of William Ayr, who died in 1875, aged twenty-four years, leaving an infant son. Mr. Scurr subsequently married Miss Dulcibel Ford, daughter of John Ford, Esq., of Sackville. They have no family. Mr. Scurr resides at Sackville and assists his father in the management of the farm.

5 John, second son of Charles and Eunice Patterson Scurr, married Miss Eliza Richardson, of Sackville. They reside at Sackville on a part of the farm his father owned, and follow farming and other industrial pursuits. They have one daughter, named Grace.

5 Annie, only daughter of Charles and Eunice Patterson Scurr, married, in 1890, Warren Cutler Anderson, son of James Anderson, of Dorchester. They reside at Dorchester. Mr. Anderson is engaged in milling and lumbering.

4 Thomas, youngest son of Benjamin and Mary Bulmer Scurr, married Elizabeth, eldest daughter of Christopher Richardson, in the year 1852. They resided on the old Scurr homestead for a number of years, and then Wm. Scurr exchanged farms with Mr. Charles Taylor, of Dorchester, to which place he removed and occupied it until his decease. Their family consisted of Mary, Charles, Christopher, Milton, Jennie, Chandler and Cassie. Mr. Scurr died in 1873, aged 49 years. His widow is still living.

5 Mary, eldest daughter of Thomas and Elizabeth Richardson Scurr, married Benjamin Chapman, farmer, of Ft. Lawrence, where they reside and have children named Ethel, Odessa and Matthew Lodge.

5 Charles, eldest son of Thomas and Elizabeth Richardson,

married Miss Alice Buck in 1887. They reside in Dorchester, farming, and have one child.

5 Jennie, second daughter of Thomas and Elizabeth Richardson Scurr, married George A. Tingley in 1885. Mr. Tingley is a farmer and only son of Thomas Tingley, Esq., of Dorchester. The children of George A. and Jennie Scurr Tingley are named Lee Anderson and Arthur Milton. The above contains the account of the posterity of Mary Bulmer and her husband, Benjamin Scurr.

3 John, third son of George and Susannah Dixon Bulmer, married Rebecca Lawrence, daughter of George Lawrence, of Sackville. They settled at Rockport, where Mr. Bulmer was engaged in milling and lumbering. He also followed his trade as a blacksmith. They had children named George, William, John, James, Ruth, Olive, Mary Ann, Laban and Nelson. Mr. Bulmer died in 1854, aged 61, and Mrs. Bulmer died in 1858.

4 George, eldest son of John and Rebecca Lawrence Bulmer, married Margaret Sutherland. They had one daughter when Mr. Bulmer died in the year 1860. The daughter grew up and married Reed Cuthbertson, of Moncton, and had one child when Mrs. Cuthbertson died in 1883, leaving an infant daughter. Mrs. Bulmer, George's widow, still survives.

4 William, second son of John and Rebecca Lawrence Bulmer, followed the sea, and became a competent shipmaster, and was familiarly called Captain William. He married an English lady named Fanny Monday, and made his residence for a time at Richibucto. They had children named John, Edward, William and Fanny. Captain William died on shipboard at sea in 1881, and his wife and children returned to England.

AND HER HUSBAND, GEORGE BULMER. 113

⁴ John, third son of John and Rebecca Lawrence Bulmer, was a cripple from childhood and died in 1858.

⁴ James, fourth son of John and Rebecca Lawrence Bulmer, married Nancy King, of Rockport, where they resided, and had four children named Sarene, William, Dora and James. Mr. Bulmer did in 1863. His widow afterwards married Jonathan Bowser.

⁵ Sarene, eldest daughter of James and Nancy King Bulmer, married James Bainbridge. They had one child, named John. Mrs. Bainbridge died in 1878.

⁵ William, eldest son of James and Nancy King Bulmer, is a shipmaster sailing out of England, where he makes his home.

⁵ Dora, second daughter of James and Nancy King Bulmer, is not married and resides at Moncton.

⁵ James, youngest son of James and Nancy King Bulmer, is not married and resides at Rockport and follows coasting.

⁴ Ruth, eldest daughter of John and Rebecca Lawrence Bulmer, married Avery White, a mechanic, and resides at Charlestown, Mass. They have children named Laura, Stanley, Winnifred, Caroline, William, and one other. Mr. White died in 1887.

⁴ Laban, fifth son of John and Rebecca Lawrence Bulmer, went when a young man to Australia, where he still resides. The other children of John and Rebecca Bulmer, viz, Olive, Mary Ann and Nelson, died of diphtheria, aged, respectively, 15, 13 and 8 years. This closes the account of John and Rebecca Lawrence Bulmer's family.

³ George, the fourth son of George and Susannah Dixon Bulmer, married Charlotte, eldest daughter of Joseph P. Rich-

ardson and widow of Otho Read, of Bay Verte. They resided at Fort Moncton for many years and followed farming and other industrial occupations. They had children named Otho Moncton, Joseph Benson, Susan, Fanny and Charlótte. Four others died in infancy. Mr. and Mrs. Bulmer removed with their family to Sackville about 1840, and settled on a portion of the Richardson estate. They were earnest and devoted Christians and lifelong members of the Methodist church. Mrs. Bulmer died in 1859 and Mr. Bulmer in 1862, aged 67.

4 Otho Moncton, eldest son of George and Charlotte R. Bulmer, married Mrs. Lydia Welling, widow of John Welling, of Shediac. They resided at Sackville and followed farming, and [had children named George Benson, Jacob Sililker, Eva Eudora, Laura Isabel, and one who died in infancy. 4 Otho M. Bulmer died in the year 1865, in the fortieth year of his age. Mrs. Bulmer still survives and was again married to a Mr. Angevine, who was lost or died at sea.

5 George Benson, eldest son of Otho M. and Lydia Welling Bulmer, is a shipmaster and is married to Miss Ruth A. Ogden, daughter of John Ogden, of Sackville. They have children named Annie Laura and Harold E. Four others died in infancy.

5 Jacob Silliker, second son of Otho M. and Lydia Welling Bulmer, is also a shipmaster, and married Miss Bertha Mills, of Rockland. They have children named Edgar Anita and Arlie, and one who died in infancy.

5 Eva Eudora, eldest daughter of Otho M. and Lydia Welling Bulmer, married Albion Gray, of Sackville, where they reside. They have children named Jennie Laura and Walter Fulton, and two others who died in infancy.

5 Laura Isabel, youngest daughter of Otho M. and Lydia Welling Bulmer, is not married, and resides with her mother and sister, Mrs. Gray.

4 Joseph Benson, second son of George and Charlotte Read Bulmer, died in the year 1849, of small pox, aged 21 years.

4 Susan, 4 Fanny and 4 Charlotte, daughters of George and Charlotte Read Bulmer, all died unmarried when about 20 years of age.

This closes the account of George Bulmer and his wife Charlotte Read Bulmer and their family.

3 Ann, third daughter of George and Susannah Dixon Bulmer, married Joseph Bowser, son of Thomas Bowser, one of the early English settlers of Sackville. Joseph Bowser was an industrious and successful farmer. In early life he took considerable interest in the militia, and was a captain in the service. He also was an active member of the Board of Commissioners of Sewers for many years, and both he and his wife were earnest and consistent members of the Methodist Church. Their family consisted of two sons and one daughter named Stephen Bamford, George Thomas, and Mary Jane, and three others died in childhood. Mrs. Bowser died in 1834, aged 39 years. Mr. Bowser subsequently married Miss Ann Bent, daughter of Vose Bent, of Fort Lawrence, who became the mother of a child who died in childhood. Mr. Bowser died in the year 1869, aged 78 years. His widow survived until 1877, when she also died at the age of 75 years.

4 Stephen Bamford, eldest son of Joseph and Ann Bulmer Bowser, died at the age of 19 years.

4 George Thomas, second son of Joseph and Ann Bulmer Bowser, married Rebecca Black, second daughter of the late

Jonathan C. Black. They reside at Sackville on the farm of his father and have no family. Mr. Bowser is an intelligent and well informed man. Owing to delicacy of health he does not actively engage in business or farming operations.

4 Mary Jane, only daughter of Joseph and Ann Bulmer Bowser, was a very intelligent, well educated and pious person, and was never married. She died in 1890, aged 63 years. This closes the account of Ann Bulmer and her husband, Joseph Bowser and family.

3 Elisabeth, fourth daughter of George and Susannah Dixon Bulmer, married Henry McLellan of Colchester County, N. S., in the year 1827. They resided in Sackville for a brief period, and then removing to Nova Scotia, finally settled at Lunenburg. They had children named Rufus Smith, Benjamin Scurr, and Susan. Mrs. McClellan died in 1870, aged 71 years, and Mr. McLellan died in 1872.

4 Rufus Smith, eldest son of Henry and Elizabeth Bulmer McLellan, married Miss Eliza Lightbody in Oct. 1878. They lived at Great Village, N. S., and had children named Frederic S. and Hugh L., one other died in infancy. Mr. Rufus S. McLellan died October 1882, aged 52 years. His widow is married to Mr. J. W. Purdy.

4 Benjamin Scurr, second son of Henry and Elizabeth Bulmer McLellan, is a mechanic and resides at Pleasant Hills, Economy, N. S. He married Miss Mary McNeil in 1866. They have children named Henry F., Aurelia E., Martha A., Fanny S., Rufus J., Harold A. and R. N. B., three of whom, viz., Aurelia E., Martha A., and Rufus J., died in childhood. Mrs. McLellan also died in November 1881, and Mr. McLellan still survives.

4 Susan, only daughter of Henry and Elizabeth Bulmer McLellan, died in 1875, unmarried.

The above contains the account of the family of Elizabeth Bulmer and her husband, Henry McLellan.

³ Isabel, fifth daughter of George and Susannah Dixon Bulmer, married James Estabrooks, son of James Estabrooks, Esq., a former reprentative of Westmoreland County, in the Provincial Parliament. They resided at Sackville and followed farming. Their children were named Susanna, Sarah Ann, George, Scurr, Milcah, William Wilson and Isabel. Mrs. Estabrooks died in 1842, aged 41 years. Mr. Estabrooks married again and had a second famlly. He died in 1874.

4 Susanna, eldest daughter of James and Isabel Estabrooks, married Edmund Kinnear, a mechanic of Sackville. Their children are Isabel, Bertha Ann, George L. Millard and Mildred, *twins*, and Andrew. One other died in infancy. Mr. Kinnear was an energetic, active and prosperons man, and accumulated a valuable property. He died in the year 1885, aged 65 years. His widow still survives.

5 Isabel, the eldest daughter of Edmund and Susan Estabrooks Kinnear, married John Gratto, a mechanic of Boston where they resided for some time. They had one son named Willie. After Mr. Gratto's death, his widow returned to Sackville and subsequently married Israel Atkinson, a mechanic who had been previously married and had some family. They have one child named Ethel.

5 Bertha Ann, second daughter of Edmund and Susan Estabrooks Kinnear, also went to Boston when a young woman, where she married James Weldon, a mechanic who died shortly after. They had no family, and Mrs. Weldon

married a second husband, a Mr. Barratt. They reside in Boston and have no family.

⁵ George L., eldest son of Edmund and Susan Estabrooks Kinnear is a painter and resides at Sackville. He married Miss Eliza Morine, of Port Medway, N. S. They have no family.

⁵ Mildred, third daughter of Edmund and Susan Estabrooks Kinnear, married Burton Richardson, a mechanic of Sackville, where they reside and have one daughter named Gertrude.

⁵ Millard, second son of Edmund and Susan Estabrooks Kinnear died at the age of 15 years.

⁵ Andrew, youngest son of Edmund and Susan Estabrooks Kinnear, is married and resides at home with his mother.

⁴ Sarah Ann, second daughter of James and Isabel Bulmer Estabrooks, married Charles G., son of the late Philip Palmer, Esq., who was also for many years a representative of the county of Westmoreland in the Provincial Parliament. Mr. Palmer resided at Sackville, and was principally occupied with his duties as Surveyor of Crown lands and farming. The children of Charles G. and Sarah Estabrooks Palmer, were named Albert, Philip, Hanford, Blair P., George, Fred and Frank and five others who died in infancy. Mrs. Palmer died in 1878, aged 55 years, and Mr. Palmer died in 1885, aged 68 years.

⁵ Albert Palmer, eldest son of Charles G. and Sarah A. Estabrooks Palmer, married Miss Jane Chase, and resides in Sackville, farming. They have children named Charles, Annie, Mary, Ella, Harvey, John and another.

⁵ Philip, second son of Charles G. and Sarah A. Estabrooks

Palmer, is a lawyer, and resides in St. John. He married Miss Eliza Bartlett. They have no family.

⁵ Hanford, third son of Charles G. and Sarah A. Estabrooks Palmer, is station agent of the I. C. Railway at Sackville. He married Miss Nancy Estabrooks, and their children are named Hattie, Annie, George, Rufus, and Elizabeth. Three others died in infancy.

⁵ George, fourth son of Charles G. and Sarah A. Estabrooks Palmer, married Miss Bessie Daizell, of St. John. They had one child who died in infancy. Mrs. Palmer died also in 1884. Mr. Palmer is an engine-driver on the I. C. Railway.

⁵ Blair, fifth son of Charles G. and Sarah A. Estabrooks Palmer, married Miss Alma Gray. They reside in Boston and have no family.

⁵ Fred, sixth son of Charles G. and Sarah A. Estabrooks Palmer is unmarried and employed on the I. C. Railway.

⁵ Frank, youngest son of Charles G., and Sarah A. Estabrooks Palmer, is a farmer residing at Sackville. He married Miss Lois Estabrooks. They have children named Charles, Bessie, and another, and one who died in infancy.

⁴ George, eldest son of James and Isabel Bulmer Estabrooks, went to Illinois, when a young man. He married Priscilla Outhouse, daughter of James Outhouse, formerly of Sackville. They have children named James, Isabel, and another. George Estabrooks died in 1870, aged 45 years.

⁴ Scurr, second son of James and Isabel Bulmer Estabrooks, also went when a young man to Illinois, and married a Miss Hall. They reside at DeKalb farming, and have children named Grant and Cora.

⁵ Grant married a Miss Hartnett, of DeKalb, and assists his father in farming.

⁵ Cora is married to Mr. James Coyne.

⁴ William Wilson, youngest son of James and Isabel Bulmer Estabrooks, is a seafaring man, engaged in the coasting trade for many years, and is commonly called Captain Wilson. He married Mary Elizabeth, daughter of H. Nelson Bulmer. Their children are Minnie Milcah, Susan J. and George W. Two others died in infancy. Mrs. Estabrooks died in 1881, aged 41 years. Mr. Estabrooks married a second time to Mary E. Welling, of Shediac. Their children are William Cecil and John Homer.

⁴ Milcah, third daughter of James and Isabel Bulmer Estabrooks, married Edwin Irons, a mechanic residing at Providence, Rhode Island. They had one child who died in infancy.

⁴ Isabel, youngest daughter of James and Isabel Bulmer Estabrooks, married Alfred Merrill. They had no family.

This closes the account of Isabel Bulmer and her husband James Estabrooks and their family.

³ Edward, the fifth son of George and Susanna Dixon Bulmer, married Asenath Kinnear, eldest daughter of Courtenay Kinnear, of Sackville. They resided a number of years upon the old homestead, and after the death of his father he removed with his family to Hopewell, Albert County, N. B. They had children named George, Susan, Solomon, Ann, Edward, Courtenay, John, Lizzie and Arthur. Mr. Bulmer died about the year 1868, aged about 65 years, and Mrs. Bulmer died about 1873.

⁴ George, the eldest son of Edward and Asenath Kinnear Bulmer, died unmarried when about 30 years of age.

AND HER HUSBAND, GEORGE BULMER.

⁴ Susan, the eldest daughter of Edward and Asenath Kinnear Bulmer, married Silas Bishop. She died soon after, leaving no children.

⁴ Solomon also died unmarried, aged about 30 years.

⁴ Ann, second daughter of Edward and Elizabeth Kinnear Bulmer, married William Rhoda. She died within a few years, leaving two children.

⁴ Edward died unmarried, aged 22 years.

⁴ Courtenay died at the age of 18 years, and ⁴ John at the age of 16 years, and ⁴ Lizzie at the age of 12 years.

⁴ Arthur, the youngest son of Edward and Asenath Kinnear Bulmer, married Miss Belle Rogers and died about 1885, leaving several children. His widow is again married.

This closes the account of Edward Bulmer and his wife Asenath Kinnear and their family.

³ H. Nelson, sixth son of George and Susanna Dixon Bulmer, married Abigail, eldest daughter of Nathan Merrill in 1832. They resided at Sackville and followed farming. Their children were Susan, Sarah Ann, Eliza Ruth, Mary Elizabeth, Hannah, James Albert, Clarinda, Nathan George, Mariner M., Elvira and Herbert. Mrs. Bulmer died in 1872, aged 58 years. Mr. Bulmer married Mrs. Robinson, widow of the late W. C. Robinson, of Bay Verte. Mrs. Bulmer the second died in 1889, Mr. Bulmer still survives a hale and vigorous man. He had the capacity for doing the work of two ordinary men, which it has been his practice to do a great part of his life.

⁴ Susan, eldest daughter of H. Nelson and Abigail Merrill Bulmer, married Wm. McKenzie, who is a section foreman on the I. C. Railroad. They reside at Moncton and have children named Annie and Alice.

⁴ Sarah Ann, second daughter of H. Nelson and Abigail Merrill Bulmer, married William Crane Bulmer, who is a machinist at Moncton as stated on page 103.

⁴ Eliza Ruth, third daughter of H. Nelson and Abigail Merril Bulmer, married Mr. William Reed, a manufacturer and merchant of Amherst, at which place they reside. They have no family.

⁴ Mary Elizabeth, fourth daughter of H. Nelson and Abigail Merrill Bulmer, married Capt. W. Wilson Estabrooks. An account of their family is given on page 120.

⁴ Hannah, fifth daughter of H. Nelson and Abigail Merrill Bulmer, died at the age of 21 years, unmarried.

⁴ James Albert, eldest son of H. Nelson and Abigail Merrill Bulmer, is a mechanic, and resides at Sackville. He married Miss Annie McConnell, a Teacher. They have a son named John W., and two daughters named Alice and Annie, and four others died in childhood and infancy.

⁴ Clarinda, sixth daughter of H. Nelson and Abigail Merrill Bulmer, married John Delaney. They lived at Sackville and had children named H. Nelson and William. Three others died in infancy. Mrs. Delaney died in 1889.

⁴ Nathan G., second son of H. Nelson and Abigail Merrill Bulmer, married Miss Jessie Ferguson. He is a mechanic, and they reside at Sackville, and have one son named Alexander and a babe. Two others died in infancy.

⁴ Mariner M., third son of H. Nelson and Abigail Merrill Bulmer, died unmarried at the age of 24 years.

⁴ Elvira, seventh daughter of H. Nelson and Abigail Merrill Bulmer, married Seth Bulmer, son of George N. Bulmer, as stated on page 100.

⁴ Herbert, youngest son of H. Nelson and Abigail Merrill Bulmer, is a mechanic and resides at Sackville. He is married to a Miss Estabrooks. They have children named Walter and Mabel. This closes the account of H. Nelson Bulmer and his wife Abigail Merrill and family.

³ William, youngest son of George and Susannah Dixon Bulmer, when a young man followed lumbering, seafaring and various other occupations. He finally settled at a village called Cherryfield, a few miles out of Moncton, where he still resides and follows farming. He too, was a man of extraordinary physical capacity, and though he has passed the four score limit is still active and vigorous. He married Miss Jane Crossman, of Moncton, and their family consists of one daughter and nine sons, as follows: Susan, William Lewis, George, James, Charles, John, Hazen, Howard, Thomas Andrew and Allan. Four others died in childhood. Mr. and Mrs. Bulmer are still hale and hearty.

⁴ Susan, eldest daughter of William and Jane C. Bulmer, married Colin McNevin, a mechanic, resfding at Moncton, and employed in the Government railway works. They have children named William, John, Angus and James, one of whom,
₅ John, is married, and all reside at Moncton.

⁴ William Lewis, eldest son of William and Jane C. Bulmer, married Catharine McQuade, of Prince Edward Island. They reside at Moncton, where Mr. Bulmer is a Section foreman on the I. C. Railway. They have children named James, Mary Jane, Margaret, Alexander, Altena, Frederic and William.

⁴ George, second son of William and Jane C..Bulmer, is married to Miss Jane Crossman, of Moncton, and resides at

Cherryfield. They have children named John, Henry, Charles, and Gordon Baxter.

⁴ James, third son of William and Jane C. Bulmer, when a young man went to the United States, and is farming in New Hampshire, and not married.

⁴ Charles, fourth son of William and Jane C. Bulmer, died at home in 1886, age 26 years.

⁴ John, fifth son of William and Jane C. Bulmer, is a farmer residing at Cherryfield. He married Miss Letitia Riley, of Shemogue. They have children named Ann, Edward, Emily, Walter, William and Rogers. All of whom are unmarried.

⁴ Hazen, sixth son of William and Jane C. Bulmer, resides at Camden in the State of Maine, and is a blacksmith by trade. He is married to a resident of that town.

⁴ Howard, seventh son of William and Jane C. Bulmer, is also a blacksmith and resides in Montana, and is married to a resident of that country.

⁴ Thomas Andrew, eighth son of William and Jane C. Bulmer, is a farmer residing at Cherryfield, and is not married.

⁴ Allan, ninth son, is at home with his parents and not married.

³ Ruth, daughter of George and Susannah Dixon Bulmer, died in childhood.

The above closes the account of the descendants of Susannah Dixon and George Bulmer, as far as the author could obtain authentic information.

Posterity of Susanna Dixon and her husband George Bulmer:

	Born.	Living.	Dead.
Children,	13	2	11
Grand Children,	98	37	61
Great Grand Children,	243	170	73
Great Great Grand Children,	239	213	26
Great Great Great Grand Children,	11	11	0
	604	433	171

GENEALOGY OF ELIZABETH DIXON AND RUFUS SMITH.

CHAPTER V.

²ELIZABETH DIXON, third daughter of Charles and Susannah Coates Dixon, was married to Dr. Rufus Smith in the year 1789. They settled at Westmoreland Point, near Fort Cumberland, at that time a centre of wealth and influence. Dr. Smith's medical practice soon attained large proportions, extending over the counties of Cumberland and Westmoreland. He belonged to one of the Loyalist families, and inherited a vigorous constitution. It is said of him that he never failed to respond promptly to the call of a patient whatever difficulties or dangers had to be encountered and overcome in the attempt to reach the patient's home. He was a kind and obliging man, ever ready to assist a neighbor or anyone who needed assistance. He represented Westmoreland county in the Assembly from 1816 to 1827, and again from 1830 to 1834. He continued the practice of his profession until within a brief period of his death, which occurred in the year 1844 in the seventy-eighth year of his age. The family of Elizabeth Dixon and her husband, Dr. Rufus Smith, consisted of

Fanny,	Born,	1790	Polly,	Born,	1792
Charles Dixon,	"	1794	William Coates,	"	1796
Mary Elizabeth,	"	1799	Matilda,	"	1802
Edward B.,	"	1805	Lucy,	"	1807
Ruth Roach,	"	1811	Diana Gay,	"	1814

One other died in infancy, and of the above named Polly and Lucy died in childhood. Mrs. Smith survived her husband fifteen years. Two of her daughters having married and being resident at Richibucto, she, with two others, removed there also, where she died in the year 1859, aged 88 years.

₃ Fanny, the eldest daughter of Rufus and Elizabeth Dixon Smith, married Martin Gay Black, of Halifax, who was the eldest son of the Rev. William Black, the widely known Pioneer Methodist preacher of the British Maratime Provinces. Martin Gay Black was a prominent merchant and business man in Halifax; a leading and active member of the Methodist church, and a liberal supporter of benevolent institutions, and highly esteemed by all classes and creeds as a Christian gentleman. The family of Martin Gay and Fanny Smith Black consisted of six sons and seven daughters, named Eliza, Rufus Smith, Alexander Anderson, Fanny, Celia, Matilda, Martin Gay, Amelia S., Louise P., William, Samuel H., Sophia and Charles, of whom the last named (₄Charles) died early.

Mrs. ³ Fanny Smith Black died in 1859, aged 68 years. Her mother, who was just 20 years her senior, died on the same day. Martin Gay Black died in 1861, aged 74 years.

⁴ Eliza and ⁴ Louise P., eldest and sixth daughters of Martin Gay and Fanny Smith Black were not married, and are deceased.

[4] Rufus Smith, eldest son of Martin Gay and Fanny Smith Black, is a medical man, who stands high in his profession. He married Miss Theresa Ferguson, daughter of John Ferguson, Esq., of Halifax. They had a family of two sons and six daughters. One of the sons died in infancy. The others are named Fanny Theresa, Mary Elizabeth, Jane Millar, John Ferguson, Louisa Pinkney, Laura Matilda and Edith Sophia.

[5] Jane Millar, third daughter of Dr. Rufus S. and Theresa Ferguson Black, married Rev. Jabez A. Rogers, a prominent minister of the Methodist church. They have had children named Charles Melville, William Arthur, Gertrude Evelyn, Eleanor Theresa, Alfred Seymour, Bertha and two others. Of the above named, Charles Melville and William Arthur, died in childhood at Amherst, in 1880, where Mr. Rogers was then stationed.

[5] John Ferguson, son of Dr. Rufus S. and Theresa Ferguson Black, is also a medical man and is not married. The other members of the family of Dr. Rufus S. and Theresa Ferguson Black are not married.

[4] Alexander Anderson, second son of Martin Gay and Fanny Smith Black, married Miss Mary Ann Leishman. They had two sons, both of whom died in childhood. Mr. Black also died in 1855, aged 42 years.

[4] Fanny, second daughter of Martin Gay and Fanny Smith Black, married James L. Matthewson, of Montreal, in 1840. They had a family named Fanny Black, John, Martin Black, Matthew Richey, Margaret Graham, Mary Elisabeth and Francis Hall, the two first named of whom died in infancy. Mr. Matthewson died in 1867, and Mrs. Matthewson died in 1877.

⁵ Martin Black, second son of James L. and Fanny Black Matthewson, married Miss Kate Grant. They had one child. Mr. Matthewson died in 1883, aged 39 years. His widow afterward married a Mr. Slaughter who is since deceased, leaving her a widow a second time.

⁵ Matthew Richey, third son of James L. and Fanny Black Matthewson, married Miss Martha Wheeler. They reside in Detroit, where Mr. M. is engaged in mercantile pursuits.

⁵ Margaret Graham, second daughter of James L. and Fanny Black Matthewson, married J. J. McLaren, Esq., a prominent lawyer of Toronto. Mrs. McLaren died in early life, and Mr. McLaren married Miss Mary Elizabeth Matthewson, sister of his former wife. They reside in Toronto and have a family of four children.

⁵ Francis Hall, youngest son of James L. and Fanny Black Matthewson, resides at Winnipeg, Manitoba, and is a banker. He married Miss Carrie Dangerfield, who died, leaving one child. ⁵ Mr. Matthewson married Miss Helen Stanton as his second wife, and they have two children.

⁴ Celia, third daughter of Martin Gay and Fanny Smith Black, married Thomas Cannon, of Liverpool, England, where they resided. Their family consists of three sons and a daughter. One of the sons died in early life. Mr. Cannon died in 1852. Mrs. Cannon afterward married a Mr. Glynn, who also died, leaving her a widow a second time.

⁴ Matilda, fourth daughter of Martin Gay and Fanny Smith Black, married Rev. Charles DeWolfe, a Methodist minister of distinguished ability, and highly esteemed by all denominations. He was appointed to many of the most important circuits, and as a pulpit and platform speaker had

few equals. He received the degree of Doctor of Divinity from Acadia College, Horton, N. S. He filled the position of Theological Professor at Mount Allison University for a number of years, and when he resigned it in 1870, became a supernumerary. The family of Rev. Charles and Matilda Black De Wolfe, consisted of one son and three daughters, two of whom died in infancy. The survivors are named Fanny and Louisa. 4 Mrs. DeWolfe died at Windsor, N. S., in 1873, aged 58 years. Dr. DeWolfe died at Horton, N. S., in 1875.

5 Fanny, eldest daughter of Rev. Charles and Matilda Black DeWolfe, married N. S. White, Esq., of Shelburne. N. S. Mr. White is a prominent lawyer and has been for some years a member of the Local Parliment. They have two sons named Thomas Howland and Charles DeWolfe.

5 Louisa, youngest daughter of Rev. Charles and Matilda Black DeWolfe, is not married.

4 Martin Gay Black, Junior, third son of Martin Gay and Fanny Smith Black, married Miss Mary Mitchell, of Chester, N. S. They had a family of five sons and three daughters. One of the sons and a daughter died in infancy and childhood. The names of the survivors are Fanny S., John B., Maria M., Henry B., William S., and Alfred C. Mr. Black for many years held a responsible position in connection with the Halifax Banking Company. He died in 1879, aged 62 years.

5 Fanny, eldest daughter of Martin G. and Mary Mitchell Black, married Alfred J. Creighton, of Halifax. They have two children named Mary Black and Alfred B. Two others died in infancy.

5 John B., eldest son of Martin G. and Mary Mitchell Black, is a resident of Londonderry, N. S.

⁵ Henry B., the second son, is in Chicago.

₅ William S. and Alfred C., the two younger sons, reside in Dartmouth, N. S., and are not married.

⁴ Amelia S., fifth daughter of Martin Gay and Fanny Smith Black, married James A. Matthewson, of Montreal, in 1847. Mr. Matthewson is a prominent business man in Montreal, and an active and zealous member of the Methodist church. The family of James A. and Amelia S. Black Matthewson, bear the names of William Black, Jessie, Henry Martyn, Fanny Smith, Rachel, Elizabeth Adams, Amelia Seabury, Samuel James, Joseph Benson, Edward Payson, James A., Ellen Hopewell, and George Herbert. Of the above named ⁵ Jessie, ⁵ Henry Martyn, ₅ Rachel, ⁵ Elizabeth Adams and ⁵ Joseph Benson died in childhood and infancy, and ⁵ Fannie Smith at the age of 12 years.

⁵ William Black, eldest son of James A. and Amelia S. Black Matthewson, married Miss Wilhelmina Ferguson, at Little Metis, Quebec, in 1873. They have children named Lawrence Adams, and Amy.

⁵ Samuel James, third son of James A. and Amelia S. Black Matthewson, married Miss Carrie Smith, daughter of the late William Howe Smith, in 1884. They have children named Frederick Howe, Amelia Evelyn, Winnifred, and James Arthur.

⁵ Edward Payson, fifth son of James A. and Amelia S. Black Matthewson, married Miss Charlotte McFarlane in 1891. They reside at Montreal. The remaining members of the family of James A. and Amelia Black Matthewson are not married.

⁴ William Black, fourth son of Martin Gay and Fanny Smith Black, never married.

⁴ Samuel H., fifth son of Martin Gay and Fanny Smith Black, married Miss Fanny E. McMurray, daughter of Rev.

John McMurray, D. D., of Windsor, N. S. Their family consists of one daughter and one son, named Nancy E. and John Henry. Mr. Black is cashier of the Halifax Banking Co.

4 Sophia, youngest daughter of Martin Gay and Fanny Smith Black, died in 1859, aged 24 years.

The above concludes the account of the families and descendants of Fanny Smith and her husband Martin Gay Black.

3 Charles D., eldest son of Doctor Rufus and Elizabeth Dixon Smith, was also a medical doctor. He married Miss Mary Elizabeth Wilson, second daughter of Benjamin Wilson, then a merchant at Dorchester. They settled at Dorchester Island. Dr. Charles, as he was familiarly called, was an excellent practitioner and universally esteemed as an honest and upright man. He was a great reader and a most entertaining and intelligent conversationalist. The family of Dr. Charles and Mary E. Wilson Smith consisted of four sons and five daughters, named Frederic, Lucy, Ellen, Fanny B., Mary, Norman, Rufus, Louisa Ann and Charles. Mrs. Smith died in 1862, aged 64 years. Dr. Charles survived his partner some 25 years, reaching the great age of 93 years. He spent the two last years of his life with his only surviving daughter at Kittery Maine, N. S., where he died in 1887.

4 Frederic, eldest son of Dr. Charles and Mary E. Wilson Smith, when a youth went to St. John, entering the employ of Messrs. Harris and Allan, where he remained for several years. He then went into business upon his own acceunt, and engaged in ship-building. He married Miss Jane Tuck, of St. John. They had children named Florence, Annie and James S. Harris.

Mr. Smith died in 1865, aged 35 years. Mrs. Smith is still living.

[5] Florence, eldest daughter of Frederic and Jane Tuck Smith, married Alban Thomas. They resided in St. John for some time and then removed to New York. They had children named Alban and Frederic, the last named of whom died in infancy. Mrs. Thomas died at Bucksport, Maine, in 1884, aged 30 years.

[5] Annie, second daugher of Frederic and James Tuck Smith, married James Douglass, a merchant at Bucksport, Maine. They have a son named John.

[5] James S. Harris, only son of Frederic and Jane Tuck Smith, died in childhood.

[4] Lucy, eldest daughter of Dr. Charles and Mary E. Wilson Smith, died unmarried in 1861, aged 40 years.

[4] Ellen, second daughter of Dr. Charles and Mary E. Wilson Smith, married Henry C. Lovell, who for a time was a business partner with James Harris & Co., at St. John. They reside at Kittery, Me., and have a son named Charles D. Smith.

[4] Fanny B., [4] Mary, and [4] Louisa Ann, daughters of [3] Dr. Charles and Mary E. Wilson Smith, all died in early life and not married.

[4] Norman, second son of Dr. Charles and Mary E. Wilson Smith, went when a young man to California. He is married and has children named Florence, Charles and Norman.

[4] Rufus, third son of Dr. Charles and Mary E. Wilson Smith, when a young man went to Australia, and is engaged in mining operations, and not married.

[4] Charles, youngest son of Dr. Charles and Mary E. Wilson

Smith, is a successful shipmaster. He married Miss Jennie Smith, a Scotch Lady, and they reside in Liverpool, England, and have a son named Gideon Palmer. This concludes the account of Charles D. and Mary E. Wilson Smith and their descendants.

³ William Coates, second son of Dr. Rufus and Elisabeth Dixon Smith, married Miss Mary B. Smith, sister of the late Thomas Smith, of Shediac. They resided for a time at St. John and also at Shediac, and finally settled at Montreal. They had children named Rufus, Eliza, William Howe, Miles B. Louisa, Diana, Edward W., Alexander A. B., and Hazen M. Mr. Smith died in 1856, aged 60 years.

⁴ Rufus, eldest son of William C. and Mary B. Smith, married Miss Eliza Trites, of Salisbury, N. B. He died in the year 1866, leaving three daughters named Blanche L., Mary C. and Ella A.

⁵ Mary C. second daughter of Rufus and Eliza Trites Smith, married Thompson Taylor and resides in Moncton.

⁴ William Howe, second son of William Coats and Mary B. Smith, married Miss Mary S. DeWolf, of Halifax. ⁴Mr. Smith died in 1890, leaving four children named William A. DeWolf, Carrie Louise, Arthur Welsford and Mary Bertha.

⁵ William A. DeWolf, eldest son of William Howe and Mary S. DeWolf Smith, married Miss Mary Smith, of Shediac, N. B. They reside in British Columbia.

⁵ Carrie Louise, eldest daughter of William Howe and Mary S. Dewolf Smith, is married to Samuel J. Matthewson, and resides in Montreal.

⁵ Mary Bertha, youngest daughter of William Howe and

Mary S. DeWolf Smith, married Fred F. Miller, of Napanee, and resides in Montreal.

⁴ Alexander A. B., fourth son of William Coates and Mary B. Smith, married Catherine Reily and resides in Chicago.

⁴ Edward W., fifth son of William Coates and Mary B. Smith, married Miss Lillie M. Davis, and they reside in Henrysburg, Quebec.

⁴ Hazen M., youngest son of William Coates and Mary B. Smith, died in 1871 unmarried.

The remainder of the family of William Coates and Mary B. Smith, viz: ⁵ Eliza, ⁵ Miles B., ⁵ Louisa and ⁵ Diana are not married.

The above contains the history of William Coates and Mary B. Smith and their decendants as far as could be obtained.

³ Mary Elizabeth and ³ Matilda, daughrers of Dr. Rufus and Elizabeth Dixon Smith, never married. Shortly after the death of their father, they with their mother removed from their old home to Richibucto, and lived near their sisters Mrs. Chandler and Mrs. Desbrisay. Here they lived in ease and quiet, enjoying the companionship of their sisters and their families, until the close of life. ³ Mary Elizabeth died in 1875, aged 75 years. ³ Matilda died in 1882, aged 80 years.

³ Edward B., youngest son of Dr. Rufus and Elizabeth Dixon Smith, married Miss Julia Webster, of Fredericton, N. B. They resided at Kingston, N. B., where Mr. Smith held the office of Registrar. They had one daughter named Louisa. Mrs. Smith died and Mr. Smith married a Mrs. Robertson, of St. John. They had no family. Mr. Smith died a few years after his second marriage,

⁴ Louisa, daughter of Edward B. and Julia Webster Smith, married Albert Lyons, of Lyons Point, on the river St. John. They have three children.

³ Ruth Roach, daughter of Dr. Rufus and Elizabeth Dixon Smith, married William B. Chandler, a lawyer residing at Richibucto, in the year 1834. Mr. Chandler held the office of Surrogate judge for Kent County. The history of the "Chandler Family" says of him: "That he was one of the first lawyers that settled in that county, and for over a quarter of a century was a most honorable and successful practitioner." The family of William B. and Ruth R. Smith Chandler, consisted of five sons and four daughters, named Rufus Smith, Mary Elizabeth, Sarah Ann, Charles Henry, Fanny Smith, Jane McCurdy, Matilda, William Botsford, and Edward Barron. Mr. Chandler died in 1856, aged 51 years, and ³ Mrs. Ruth R. Chandler died in 1868, aged 57 years.

⁴ Rufus Smith, eldest son of William B. and Ruth R. Smith Chandler, is a merchant residing at Dalhousie, N. B. He married Miss Mary Barbarie in 1862. They had two children named Florence Evelyn, and Ruth Roach Smith. Mrs. Chandler died in 1868, aged 30 years. ⁴ Mr. Chandler married Miss Euphemia A. McBeath for a second wife in 1873. They had children named Edgar and Mary. ⁵ Mary died in 1888, aged 12 years. Mrs. Chandler died in 1885, aged 50 years.

⁴ Mary Elizabeth, eldest daughter of Wm. B. and Ruth R. Smith Chandler, married Richard B. Haddow, merchant of Miramichi. They had five children, four of whom died in childhood. The survivor is named ⁵ Mary Emily Fanny, and resides at Newcastle, N. B.

⁴ Sarah Ann, second daughter of William B. and Ruth R.

Smith Chandler, married Thomas W. Dibblee in 1863. Mr. Dibblee was a lawyer and resided at Richibucto. They had three children named William Chandler, George Jarvis and Lewis, the last named of whom died in childhood. Mr. Dibblee died in 1870.

⁵ William Chandler Dibblee, son of Thomas W. and Sarah A. Chandler Dibblee, is a Telegraph Operator in California.

⁵ George Jarvis Dibblee is clerk in an Insurance office in Toronto.

⁴ Charles Henry, second son of William B. and Ruth R. Smith Chandler, was educated at Mount Allison College. He studied law with his father, and also in the office of the present Judge Wetmore at St. John, and was admitted to the Bar in 1863. He held the office of Law Librarian and clerk of the Police Court of St. John. He married Miss A. B. Doan, daughter of Captain J. W. Doan. They had one child named ⁵ Gertrude Louise. ⁴ Mr. Chandler died in 1881, aged 41 years.

⁴ Fanny Smith, third daughter of William B. and Ruth R. Smith Chandler is not married, and resides at Dorchester in the family of the late Governor Chandler.

⁴ Jane McCurdy, fourth daughter of William B. and Ruth R. Smith Chandler, married her cousin Rufus S. Desbrisay. They had one child named Percy Brisaif. Mrs. Desbrisay died at Greenock, Scotland, in 1870, aged 22 years.

⁴ Matilda, fifth daughter of William B. and Ruth R. Smith Chandler, married Mr. Robert Caie, of Richibucto. They had one child who died in infancy. Mrs. Caie died in 1870, aged 24 years.

⁴ William Botsford, third son of William B. and Ruth R. Smith Chandler, and also his brother, ⁴ Edward Barron Chan-

dler, were educated at King's College, Windsor, N. S., and reside at Collingwood, Ontario. The above comprises the account of the family of Ruth Roach Smith and her husband William B. Chandler.

³ Diana Gay, youngest daughter of Dr. Rufus and Elisabeth Dixon Smith, married Lestock P. W. Desbrisay, a leading merchant and extensive mill and ship owner residing at Richibucto. Mr. Desbrisay was a man of much energy and conducted a large business. He represented the County a number of years in the Provincial Parliament with ability. The family of Mr. Desbrisay consisted of five sons and three daughters named Rufus Smith, Lucy Wright, Mary Smith, Theophilus, Lestock P. Wilson, George Wright, Elisabeth, and Thomas De La Cour. Mr. Desbrisay died at Richibucto in December 1872, and Mrs. Desbrisay died in February 1877, aged 62 years.

⁴ Rufus Smith. eldest son of Lestock P. W. and Diana G. Smith Destrisay, married Jane McCurdy, fourth daughter of William B. and Ruth R. Smith Chand,er, who died at Greenock as previously stated. Rufus S. Desbrisay died in January 1880, aged 37 years.

⁴ Lucy Wright Desbrisay is married.

⁴ Mary Smith Desbrisay died in infancy.

⁴ Lestock P. W., third son of Lestock P. W. and Diana G. Smith Desbrisay is married and resides at Calgarry.

⁴ Elizabeth, third daughter of L. P. W. and Diana G. Smith Desbrisay, married Frank Hazard, a Barrister, of Charlottetown, Prince Edwards Island, where they reside.

⁴ Thomas De La Cour, youngest son of Lestock P. W. and Diana C. Smith Desbrisay, died in 1883.

AND RUFUS SMITH. 139

The foregoing comprises the account of the family of Diana G. Smith and her husband Lestock P. W. Desbrisay.

Posterity of Elizabeth Dixon and her husband Dr. Rufus Smith.

	Born.	Living.	Dead.
Children	11	0	11
Grand Children	48	26	22
Great Grand Children	81	55	26
Great Great Grand Children	32	27	5
	172	108	64

GENEALOGY OF RUTH DIXON AND THOMAS ROACH.

CHAPTER VI.

² RUTH DIXON, fourth daughter of Charles and Susannah Coates Dixon, married Thomas Roach in the year 1793. Mr. and Mrs. Roach settled at Fort Lawrence where Mr. Roach owned a large and valuable property. He was also engaged in Merchandise and subsequently in shipbuilding. Mr. Roach was elected to the Provincial Parliment in 1799 and occupied a seat in that body until 1826, having been elected five times in succession. Mr. Roach was a Methodist Local Preacher of more than ordinary ability and a liberal supporter of Methodist and benevolent institutions. The family of Thomas and Ruth Dixon Roach consisted of the following, viz:

John,	Born,	1794	Susannah D.,	Born,	1795
Jean,	"	1797	Charles D.,	"	1800
Mary,	"	1802	Thomas,	"	1805
Edward,	"	1807			

Mrs. Roach died in March 1810, in the 38th year of her age. In a memoir of her, written by her husband, it is stated that about one week previous to her death she was taken ill and complained of a severe pain in her side, and that medical aid was not obtained for about three days. When her brother-in-law, Dr. Rufus Smith, was called, who

GENEALOGY OF RUTH DIXON 141

bled her on the occasion of his first visit, which was on Sunday and again on Monday, and again on Tuesday, and that Mrs. Roach died the folowing Thursday. ` Doubtless the medical treatment she received would be very unfavorably regarded at the present day, yet there is no room to doubt that Dr. Smith did all in his power to arrest the progress of the disease and save the life of one so greatly beloved and esteemed, with whom he and his family were so nearly connected. Mr. Roach says of her that she was a devoted Christian woman and died in the faith of the Gospel.

Mr. Roach was subsequently married, first, to a widow lady, Mrs. Sarah Allan, and after her death, to a Miss Mary Dickson of Onslow, N. S., and after her decease to a Miss Charlotte Wells, who survived him several years. None of the three last wives left children. Mr. Roach died in 1833, aged 65 years.

3 John, eldest son of Thomas and Ruth Dixon Roach, married Miss Sarah A. Dixon, of Onslow, in January 1824. They resided at Meccan, where he owned a large and valuable farm. Mr. Roach was a man of strict integrity, a zealous and devoted member and liberal supporter of the Methodist Church, and a highly respected member of the community in which he lived. The family of John and Sarah A. Dixon Roach, consisted of five sons and two daughters named L. Dickson, Ruth R., Thomas, Robert D., Edward DeWolfe, John E., and James T. J., who died in childhood. Mr. Roach died in the year 1862, aged 67 years, and Mrs. Roach survived her husband about five years.

4 L. Dickson, eldest daughter of John and Sarah A. Dickson Roach, married William Wellington Blair, a farmer of Truro,

N. S. Their family consisted of six daughters and three sons, named Eliza, Florence, Laura, Fanny, Hibbard, Louis, Roland, Josephine and Susan C. Mrs. Blair died in 1885 aged 60 years.

⁵ Eliza, eldest daughter of William W. and L. Dickson Roach Blair, married William Embree a farmer of Amherst. They have one child named Edith.

⁵ Florence, second daughter of William W. and L. Dickson Roach Blair, married Dr. Chipman, of Grand Pre. They have one child named Laura Annie.

⁵ Laura, third daughter of William W. and L. Dickson Roach Blair, married Dr. Chipman of Grand Pre. They had one child named Robert Somerville. Mrs. Chipman died soon after the birth of her child, and Mr. Chipman married her sister ⁵ Florence as his second wife as before stated. The remainder of the family of Mr. Blair and L. Dickson Roach are not married.

⁴ Ruth R., second daughter of John and Sarah A. Dickson Roach, is not married. For many years she has lived with her brother, Robert D., and assisted him in his duties of Postmaster and Station agent at Meccan.

⁴ Thomas, eldest son of John and Sarah A. Dickson Roach, is a farmer residing at Meccan. He married Miss Susan Bishop, of Onslow, and they have children named Frank Edwin, Emily, John and Walter. The last named of whom died in childhood. Mr. and Mrs. Roach are active members of the Methodist church.

⁴ Robert D., second son of John and Sarah A. Dickson Roach, is not married, and resides at Meccan, where he has for

many years filled the office of Postmaster and Station agent as before stated.

⁴ Elisha De Wolfe, third son of John and Sarah A. Dickson Roach, is a medical Doctor residing at Tatamagouche, N. S. He married Miss Sophia McKeen. They had children named Fanny and John, both of whom died in childhood. Mrs. Roach died in 1880.

⁴ John E., fourth son of John and Sarah A. Dickson Roach, is a farmer residing at Meccan. He married Miss Mary Dunlap, of Truro. They had a son named Clinton. Mrs. Roach died in 1880, and Mr. Roach afterward married Miss Sarah Harrison, of Meccan. They have children named Sophia, Bessie and Lavinia. Mr. Roach is an active and leading man in the community where he resides.

The account of the family of John Roach here closes.

³ Susan D., eldest daughter of Thomas and Ruth Dixon Roach, married William Crane in 1813. William Crane was a son of Colonel Crane, of Horton, N. S., and at the time of his marriage had been in business at Sackville several years.

Mr. Crane was a very active, enterprising man, possessing a remarkable capacity for business, and his business grew so rapidly that he was obliged to seek assistance, and he induced Charles F. Allison, who was then a clerk for Mr. Ratchford at Parrsboro, to become his partner, and soon afterward Joseph F. Allison was employed as a clerk and subsequently became partner also; and the firm of Crane & Allisons was known as among the most substantial business houses in the Provinces. In the year 1840, Charles F. Allison retired from the firm and devoted his time and a large portion of his fortune to the erection of the Mount Allison Weslyan Academy. A few years later, Joseph F. Allison also retired from the firm. Mr. Crane continued in business until his death. Mr. Crane early became interested in politics, and in 1824 was elected to the Assembly to fill a vacancy caused by the death of Benjamin Wilson, one of the representatives of the county of Westmoreland. Mr. Crane represented the county continuously from 1824 to 1842, when he was appointed to a seat in the Legislative Council, which he held until 1850, when he was again elected to the Assembly, and was a second time elected speaker of that body. Mr. Crane was on two occasions a delegate to the English Government to arrange the settlement of several important matters affecting the interests of the Province, and received the unanimous thanks of the Legislature for the great ability he displayed in the discharge of the important duties entrusted to him. The family of William and Susan D. Roach Crane consisted of one daughter named Ruth. Mrs. Crane died in 1830, deeply regretted by all who knew her. Several years later Mr. Crane married Miss Eliza Wood, and they had a family of four daughters and a son.

Mr. Crane was severely afflicted with rheumatism for a number of years, and subject to great physical suffering, which he endured with remarkable patience and fortitude. He died at Fredericton, N. B. while attending to his Legislative duties, on the 31st of March, 1853, in the 69th year of his age.

[4] Ruth, only daughter of William and Susannah D. Roach Crane, married Edward Cogswell, formerly of Horton, N. S., but who for several years previous to his marriage, was chief business clerk for Mr. Crane. The marriage took place in 1850. Their family consists of William C., Arthur E., Susan E., and Minnie Gordon, all of whom are unmarried. Mr. Cogswell died

in 1874 aged 60 years. Mr. Cogswell is again married as will appear in Chapter VIII.

[3] Jean, second daughter of Thomas and Ruth Dixon Roach, married Michael Gordon in the year 1817. They settled at Fort Lawrence. Mr. Gordon held the office of Collector of Customs for a long period, and was also an active and leading Magistrate. The family of Michael and Jean Roach Gordon, consisted of seven sons and three daughters, named Ruth Roach, Thomas Roach, Michael Frederic, William Crane, Edward F., Susan C., George B., N. Jefferson, Allan, and Susan Jane. Mr. Gordon died in 1862, aged 69 years. Mrs. Gordon died in 1858, aged 60 years.

[4] Ruth Roach, eldest daughter of Michael and Jean Roach Gordon, married Thomas Woodman, son of an English Gentleman who came with his family to Cumberland about the year 1840, and for some time resided at Fort Cumberland. Mr. and Mrs. Thomas Woodman settled at Moncton where Mr. Woodman taught for some years a superior school. Their family consisted of six sons and a daughter, named Gordon, Eliza, Thomas, John, George, Charles and Edward. Mrs. Woodman died recently at Moncton in the 73d year of her age. Mr. Woodman died at Tangier, N. S. in 1876.

[5] Gordon, the eldest son of Thomas and Ruth Roach Gordon Woodman, was drowned in 1861, aged 17 years.

[5] Eliza, only daughter of Thomas and Ruth R. Gordon Woodman, died in 1865, aged 19 years.

[5] Thomas, second son of Thomas and Ruth R. Gordon Woodman, is a mechanic residing at or near Boston. He married Miss Louisa Higgins, and they have four children.

[5] John, third son of Thomas and Ruth R. Gordon Wood-

man, is also a mechanic residing at Boston. He married Miss Agnes Carter, and they have two children.

⁵ George, fourth son of Thomas and Ruth R. Gordon Woodman, is a printer residing at Moncton. He married Miss Isabella McQuarrie, and they had a child named Florence. Mrs. Woodman died, and Mr. Woodman married for his second wife, Miss Elospay Mitchell, and they have children named Jane, George and Hattie.

⁵ Charles, fifth son of Thomas and Ruth R. Gordon Woodman, is an Engineer residing in Boston, unmarried.

₅ Edward, youngest son of Thomas and Ruth R. Gordon Woodman, is an electrician, residing at Boston. He married Miss Jennie McDonald, and they have one child.

⁴ Thomas R. Gordon, eldest son of Michael and Jean Roach Gordon, in early life became a clerk in the store of W. Tisdale and Son at St. John. In due time he commenced business for himself. He married Miss Mary A. Gaynor, of St. John. They had two sons named Charles and Frank. Mr. Gordon removed with his family to the United States, many years since and settled at Brooklyn, New York, where he and his sons still reside. Mrs. Gordon died several years since.

⁵ Charles, eldest son of Thomas R. and Mary A. Gaynor Gordon, is married and resides at Brooklyn.

⁴ Michael Frederic, second son of Michael and Jean Roach Gordon, also went when a youth to St. John, where he was a clerk for some years. He married Miss Abbie Hawes and in a few years after, they went to Australia. They had two children when they left St. John. Mr. Gordon is principal Customs officer at Geelong, Australia.

⁴ William Crane, third son of Michael and Jean Roach

Gordon, is a painter. He is not married and resides at Port Elgin, N. B.

⁴ Susan C., second daughter of Michael and Jean Roach Gordon, died in childhood.

⁴ Edward F., fourth son of Michael and Jean Roach Gordon, also followed the occupation of a Clerk. He married Miss Albina Hartt, of Fredericton. Owing to failure of health he went to Chicago where he died suddenly, leaving a widow who has married again.

⁴ George B., fifth son of Michael and Jean Roach Gordon, was lost at sea when a young man and unmarried.

⁴ N. Jefferson, sixth son of Michael and Jean Roach Gordon, is a farmer residing at Fort Lawrence upon the old homestead of his Father. He married Miss Harriet Gordon of Windsor, N. S. They have no family.

⁴ Allan, seventh son of Michael and Jean Roach Gordon, died of consumption, aged 30 years. He was not married.

⁴ Susan Jane, youngest child of of Michael and Jean Roach Gordon, married Alexander Allan. They resided in Portland, Maine. They had no family. Mrs. Allan died in 1888, aged 54 years.

The foregoing account of the family of Jean Roach and her husband, Michael Gordon, is as complete as could be obtained.

³ Charles D., second son of Thomas and Ruth Dixon Roach, when a young man studied law, but did not engage in the practice of that profession. He followed farming at Westmoreland and afterward removed to Amherst, where he followed farming and land surveying. He married Miss Rebecca Carritt in the year 1825. Their children were named Thomas, Eleanor,

William, John C., Edward, Ruth, Frederic, Marshall and Botsford Allison. One other died in infancy. Charles D. Roach died in the year 1880, aged 79 years, and Mrs. Roach died in 1885.

4 Thomas, the eldest son of Charles D. and Rebecca C. Roach, is a farmer residing at Amherst. He married Miss Eliza Smith, daughter of James Smith, Esq., of Fort Lawrence. They have children named Hibbert, James and Annie.

5 Hibbert, eldest son of Thomas and Eliza Smith Roach, is married and has two children. He resides in New York.

5 James, second son of Thomas and Eliza Smith Roach is a farmer residing at Salem near Amherst. He married Miss Francis Greeno, as stated on page 21.

5 Annie, only daughter of Thomas and Eliza Smith Roach, resides at home and is not married.

4 Eleanor, eldest daughter of Charles D. and Rebecca C. Roach, died in 1863, aged 34 years, unmarried.

4 William, second son of Charles D. and Rebecca C. Roach, is a mechanic and resides at Windsor, N. S. He married Miss Harriet Atkinson, of Shediac, N. B. They have children named William, Clara, Adelaide, Ellen Ruth, George, Minnie, Frank and Frederic. Of the above named, 5William and 5 Clara are married.

4 John C., third son of Charles D. and Rebecca C. Roach, died unmarried in 1866, aged 34 years.

4 Edward, fourth son of Charles D. and Rebecca C. Roach, died in 1861, unmarried, aged 26 years.

4 Ruth, second daughter of Charles D. and Rebecca C. Roach, married Charles Copp, of Westmoreland, N. B. They lived at Amherst. They had one child who died in infancy. Mrs. Copp died in 1864, aged 27 years.

⁴ Fred, fifth son of Charles D. and Rebecca C. Roach, is a mechanic, and resides at Dartmouth, N. S. He married a Miss Thomas, of Waverly, N. S. Their family consists of two daughters and a son. Mrs. Roach died in 1884.

⁴ Marshall, sixth son of Charles D. and Rebecca C. Roach, married Miss Abbie Hicks, of Maine. They reside in Chicago, and their children are named Ida and Ada (twins), Flossie and another, a boy. Mr. Roach is a mechanic.

⁴ Botsford Allison, youngest son of Charles D. and Rebecca C. Roach, is a farmer residing at Amherst on the homestead farm of his Father. He married Miss Annie Treen, of Wallace, N. S. Their children are named Laura, Charles, Ellen, Walter, Stanley, Mary, Frank and Allison, three of whom, viz., Laura, Ellen and Mary died in childhood.

The account of the family of Charles D. Roach and Rebecca Carritt here closes.

³ Mary, the third daughter of Thomas and Ruth Dixon Roach, died in childhood.

³ Thomas Roach, third son of Thomas and Ruth Dixon Roach, was lame from his infancy. He resided for a time after the death of his father on the old homestead at Fort Lawrence. He married Miss Adelia Purdy. They had no family. Mrs. Roach died in 1844. Mr. Roach sold out his property and removed to St. John, N. B. He married for his second wife Miss Lizzie Ross. Mr. Roach was salesman in the store of James Harris & Co. for a number of years. Tne family consisted of one son named James Harris. Mr. Roach died in 1876, aged 72 years. His widow and son reside in Augusta, Maine.

³ Edward, youngest son of Thomas and Ruth Dixon Roach, married Miss Margaret Liddell, of Halifax, N. S. They resided at Picton, N. S., where Mr. Roach practiced law. Their family consisted of eight children, four of whom died in childhood. The survivors are named Margaret, Bessie, John and Robert. Mr. Roach died in 1878, aged 71 years. Mrs. Roach still survives.

⁴ Margaret, eldest daughter of Edward and Margaret Liddell Roach, married George Carritt of New Glasgow, N. S., where Mr. Carritt held a situation in the Albion Coal Mining Co. Their children were named Maud, Henrietta, and Edward. Mrs. Carritt died in 1878, and Mr. Carritt died in 1884.

⁴ Bessie, second daughter of Edward and Margaret Liddell Roach, married Thomas Stabb, a merchant of St. Johns, Newfoundland. They have two sons and a daughter, named Edward, Arthur and Mabel. Mrs. Stabb died in 1887, aged 49 years.

⁵ Edward, eldest son of Thomas and Bessie Roach Stabb, married a Miss Mott, of Halifax.

⁵ Arthur and ⁵ Mabel Stabb are not married.

⁴ John, eldest son of Edward and Margaret Liddell Roach, married Miss Sarah Royal, of Sunderland, England. They reside at Fort Lawrence and have children named Leah and Hattie.

⁴ Robert, the youngest son of Edward and Margaret Liddell Roach, is not married, and his place of residence is a portion of the time in Newfoundland and the residue in Nova Scotia.

The foregoing completes the account of the family of Ruth Dixon and Thomas Roach.

Posterity of Ruth Dixon and Thomas Roach.

	Born.	Living.	Dead.
Children	7	0	7
Grand Children	37	20	17
Great Grand Children	68	57	11
Great Great Grand Children	15	15	0
Totals,	127	92	35

GENEALOGY OF MARTHA DIXON AND BENJAMIN WILSON.

CHAPTER VII.

²MARTHA, youngest daughter of Charles and Susanna Coates Dixon, married the Rev. Benjamin Wilson in 1793. Mr. Wilson was a native of Virginia, and appointed by one of the American Conferences, at the request of Bishop Black, to labor in the Provinces. He came to the Cumberland Circuit early in the year 1793. In 1795 he was sent to St. John. He occupied several other circuits in New Brunswick and Nova Scotia, remaining in the work of the ministry about ten years, when he decided to locate. His father-in-law, Mr. Dixon, supplied him with the capital to commence merchandise at Dorchester, and a short time after permitted his son William C., to enter as a partner into the business, which was conducted until about 1820 in the name of Wilson & Dixon. During the latter part of this partnership term, the firm experienced heavy losses in their lumbering operations, and through the failure, or dishonesty, of an agent in England. Mr. Wilson very soon became a prominent man in the community and in 1820 was elected one of the representatives for Westmoreland County in the Provincial Parliament. Mr. Wilson's death occurred September 20th, 1824. While in the act of crossing the Straits of Northumberland in a small

GENEALOGY OF MARTHA DIXON 153

schooner laden with salt, commanded by Capt. Samuel Cornwall, through the inclemency of the weather or other causes, the vessel, cargo and all on board were lost. [2] Mrs. Wilson survived her husband about twenty-five years, and died in 1849, aged 74 years.

The family of [2] Martha Dixon and her husband Benjamin Wilson, bore the following names:
Susanna, born Aug., 1795.   Mary Elisabeth, born May, 1798
Martha, born May, 1804.   Jane Ruth, born March, 1806.
Benjamin, born Mar. 1808.   Fanny Black, born June, 1810.
Louisa Ann, born Jun., 1812.   Charles, born May, 1815.
Hannah Caroline, born July, 1819.

Three others, viz. Joseph, Ann and Edward, died in childhood and infancy.

[3] Susanna Wilson, eldest daughter of Benjamin and Martha Dixon Wilson, married James Sayre, of Dorchester. James Sayre, was the eldest son of Mr. Sayre, who was Sheriff of Westmoreland County for a long time. James Sayre was appointed Deputy Sheriff and acted in that capacity the greater part of his life. The family of James and Susanna Wilson Sayre, consisted of the following, viz: Fanny Howard, John E., Benjamin Wilson, James F., William Henry, Charles, Jane Ruth, and one who died in childhood.

[4] Fanny Howard, eldest daughter of James and Susanna Wilson Sayre, died unmarried aged thirty years.

[4] John E., eldest son of James and Susanna Wilson Sayre, was a machinist and car builder, in the employ of his uncle James Harris, where he learned the business. He married Miss Julia Travis, of St. John. They had children named Lizzie, Frederic, and Julia Hanford. Mrs. Sayre died about 1870.

Mr. Sayre married for his second wife Miss McCallum of St. John. Mr. Sayre died in 1877, aged 50 years. His widow is still living.

⁵ Lizzie and ⁵ Julia Hanford, daughters of John E. and Julia Travis Sayre died in early life unmarried.

⁵ Frederic, only son of John E. and Julia Travis Sayre, married Miss Holly, of Portland. They had one child. Mrs. Sayre died in 1889. Mr. Sayre is again married.

₄ Benjamin Wilson, second son of James and Susanna Wilson Sayre, was a mechanic. He married Miss Rebecca Davidson of River Philip, N. S., where they resided. Mr. Sayre was engaged in merchandise and milling. They had children named Clifford, Susan, Charles John, Julia, Robert, and two others who died in childhood.

⁴ Mr. Sayre died in 1877. His widow still survives and resides at Moncton.

⁵ Clifford, eldest son of Benjamin W. and Rebecca Davidson Sayre, was a medical doctor residing at Moncton, where he had a good practice. He married Mrs. Williams, a widow lady of Parrsboro. ₅ Dr. Sayre died recently.

⁵ Susan, eldest daughter of Benjamin W. and Rebecca Davidson Sayre, married Mr. Hennigar Blenkhorn of Canning, N. S., where they reside. They have children named Clifford Sayre, Stanley, and a babe.

⁵ Charles, second son of Benjamin W. and Rebecca Davidson Sayre, is a mechanic. He married Miss Ruddick, of Sussex, N. B. They reside in Washington State.

⁵ John, third son of Benjamin W. and Rebecca Davidson Sayre, is in a drug store at Amherst and not married.

⁵ Julia, second daughter of Benjamin W. and Rebecca Davidson Sayre, is a Teacher, and not married.

⁵ Robert, the youngest son, resides with his Mother at Moncton.

⁴ James F., third son of James and Susanna Wilson Sayre is a superior machinist, and has a position next to that of the Mechanical Superintendent in the Government Railway Works at Moncton, where he resides. He married Miss Martha Gray, of St. John, who died in 1881, leaving no issue. Mr. Sayre married for a second wife Miss Eliza Stewart of St. Stephen, N. B. They have no family.

⁴ William Henry, fourth son of James and Susanna Wilson Sayre, is also a mechanic and resides at Amesbury, Mass., where he married Miss Doubtful Rowell. They have a daughter named Susanna.

⁴ Charles, fifth son of James and Susanna Wilson Sayre, when a young man went to the United States, and became an officer in the Northern Army, and was killed in the late war.

⁴ Jane Ruth, youngest daughter of James and Susanna Wilson Sayre, married Leonard Crear. bookkeeper of St. John, where they lived several years, and then removed to Boston. Their children are Charles, Minnie, Emily and Maud.

This closes the account of the family of Susanna Wilson and her husband, James Sayre.

³ Mary Elizabeth Wilson, second daughter of Benjamin and Martha Dixon Wilson, married Dr. Charles Smith, whose history is given in Chapter V.

³ Martha Wilson, third daughter of Benjamin and Martha Dixon Wilson, married Andrew Weldon, son of John Weldon, of Dorchester. This marriage took place about the year 1822.

They resided at Dorchester. Mr. Weldon was a Coroner and also Register of Deeds and Wills. The family of Andrew and Martha Wilson Weldon consisted of four sons and four daughters, named William John, Martha Ann, Benjamin Wilson, Mary Elizabeth, James Stuart, Fannie Louisa, Charles W. and Emma J. Andrew Weldon died in 1863, aged 61 years and 3 Mrs. Weldon died in 1887, aged 83 years.

4 William John, eldest son of Andrew and Martha Wilson Weldon, was a mechanic and was also engaged in farming a few years; after which he removed to Shediac, where he went into the hotel business. From thence he removed to Moncton and continued the hotel business there. He married Miss Mary J. Hickman in 1849. Their children were named James D., Martha A., William J., Adelaide H , Charles C., Edward D. and Mary E. Mr. Weldon died at Moncton in 1883, aged 60 years. Mrs. Weldon still survives.

5 James D., eldest son of William J. and Mary J. Hickman Weldon, resides at Shediac and is in the hotel business. He married Miss Burns, of Shediac. They have children named Adelaide L., Mary, Minnie, Haliburton and Elsie.

5 Martha A., eldest daughter of William J. and Mary J. Hickman Weldon, married Thomas Geddes, clerk. They had a child who died in infancy. Mr. Geddes died about a year after his marriage. His widow is married to Mr. George Ryan, Postal clerk. They reside at Moncton and have a daughter named Mary. Another child of theirs died in infancy.

5 William J., second son of William J. and Mary J. Hickman Weldon, is a Postal clerk, residing at Moncton. He married Miss Laura Purdy, of Westchester, N. S. They have four

children, named William, Laura Bell, Charles Hickman and Adelaide.

⁵ Adelaide H., second daughter of William J. and Mary J. Hickman Weldon, died unmarried, aged 22 years.

⁵ Charles C., third son of William J. and Mary J. Hickman Weldon, is a druggist, residing in British Columbia, and is not married.

⁵ Edward D., fourth son of William J. and Mary J. Hickman Weldon, is a bookkeeper, and resides in New York. He married a Miss Ford. They had a son who died in infancy.

⁵ Mary E., youngest daughter of William J. and Mary J. Hickman Weldon, is married to Wm. Gordon Blair, of Chatham, N. B.

⁴ Martha Ann, eldest daughter of Andrew and Martha Wilson Weldon, married A. L. Palmer, Esq., in 1849. Mr. Palmer was then a prominent barrister residing at Dorchester, where he practiced his profession successfully for many years. He removed to St. John about 1868, where he obtained a large and lucrative practice. He represented St. John County, in the Parliament of Canada for some years, and was appointed Judge in Equity about 1879. The family of Judge and Martha Weldon Palmer consisted of two sons and a daughter, named Arthur Lockwood, Fanny E., and Charles Arthur.

⁴ Mrs. Palmer, who was a universally esteemed and exemplary christian lady, died in 1882, aged 57 years, regretted by all. Judge Palmer married a second time. His present wife was Miss Troop of St. John.

⁵ Arthur Lockwood, eldest son of Judge and Martha A. Weldon Palmer, died in childhood.

⁵ Fanny E., only daughter of Judge and Martha A. Weldon

Palmer, is not married. She resides at St John and is a very active and zealous Christian worker, devoting both time and means to the promotion of christian and charitable enterprises.

⁵ Charles A., youngest son of Judge and Martha A. Weldon' Palmer, is a prominent lawyer of St. John. He married Miss Ada P. Sancton, and their children are named Arthur L. and George S.

⁴ Benjamin Wilson, second son of Andrew and Martha Wilson Weldon, married Miss Emmeline Hicks, of Dorchester, in 1849. They settled at Bathurst, N. B. Mr. Weldon was appointed Sheriff of the County of Gloucester, an office he held until his decease. The family of B. Wilson and Emmeline Hicks Weldon consisted of six sons and five daughters, named Charles Edward, James S., Sophia M., Emma J., Arthur, Minnie, John, Maud M., Frederic W., Andrew W., and Ella. ⁴ Mr. B. Wilson Weldon died in 1872. Mrs. Weldon was again married, first to a Mr. Vanstone, and after his death to a Mr. Sewell of Wisconsin.

⁵ Charles Edward, eldest son of B. Wilson and Emmeline Hicks Weldon, married a Miss Weldon, of Hillsborough, N. B., where they reside.

⁵ James S., second son of B. Wilson and Emmeline Hicks Weldon, married a Miss Atkinson of Amherst, N. S. They reside in Wisconsin and have one daughter.

⁵ Sophia M., eldest daughter of B. Wilson and Emmeline Hicks Weldon, married Frank Allison, eldest son of Joseph F. Allison, Esq., late of Sackville. They reside at Elkhorn, Wis., and have two children.

⁵ Emma J., second daughter of B. Wilson and Emmeline

Hicks Weldon, married a Mr. Curtiss, a farmer of Wisconsin, where they reside. They have two children, a son and a daughter.

₅ Minnie, third daughter of B. Wilson and Emmeline Hicks Weldon, married a Mr. Marr, of Pennsylvania. They had a son and a daughter. Mrs. ⁵ Marr died in 1887, aged 25 years.

₅ Arthur, third son of B. Wilson and Emmeline Hicks Weldon, resides in Wisconsin, unmarried.

⁵ John, fourth son of B. Wilson and Emmeline Hicks Weldon, is farming in Wisconsin, and is married and has one child.

⁵ Maud M., fourth daughter of B. Wilson and Emmeline Hicks Weldon, is also married and lives in Wisconsin.

⁵ Fred W., fifth son of B. Wilson and Emmeline Hicks Weldon, married a Miss Atcheson, of Newcastle, N. B. They reside at Victoria, British Columbia, where Mr. Weldon is conductor on a railway.

₅ Andrew W., youngest son of B. Wilson and Emmeline Hicks Weldon, was a brakeman on a railway in the Canadian Northwest, and was killed by a fall from the train when he was about 18 years of age.

₅ Ella, youngest daughter of B. Wilson and Emmeline Hicks Weldon, married Percy F. Gabe, of Missouri, where they reside.

⁴ Mary Elizabeth, second daughter of Andrew and Martha Wilson Weldon, married J. E. Upham, merchant of Kings County, N. B., in 1848. They had children named Andrew W., Kate E., Charles W. and Fanny L. Mrs. Upham died in 1859, aged 32 years, and Mr. Upham died about two years later.

⁵ Andrew W., eldest son of J. E. and Mary E. Weldon Upham, is a shipmaster. He married Miss Mary E. Wilson, daughter of the late Doctor Wilson, of Dorchester. They reside at St. John and have two children, named Ellen W. and Charles E.

⁵ Kate E., eldest daughter of J. E. and Mary E. ·Weldon Upham, married William H. Nevius, of the firm of P. I. Nevius and Sons, of New York. They have a daughter named Frances Joy. Another child died in infancy.

⁵ Charles W., second son of J. E. and Mary E. Weldon Upham, was a shipmaster. He married Miss Eliza Fowler, of St. John. They had a child named Winnifred W. Capt. Upham died in 1887, aged 33 years. His widow and son reside at St. John.

⁵ Fanny L., second daughter of J. E. and Mary E. Weldon Upham, married Charles S. Harding, a merchant of St. John. They have two children named Florence W. and J. Wentworth.

⁴ James Stuart, third son of Andrew and Martha Wilson Weldon, when a young man went to Australia, where he still resides, unmarried.

⁴ Fanny L., third daughter of Andrew and Martha Wilson Weldon, married Thomas D. Henderson, merchant of St. John, in 1857. Their children are named Emma V., Mary U., Martin G. B., Charles W., Fanny E., Stanley H. and Thomas Aubrey. The two last named died in childhood.

⁵ Emma V., eldest daughter of Thomas D. and Fanny L. Weldon Henderson, married William Smith, clerk, of St. John, where they reside and have a son named Stanley M.

⁴ Charles W., youngest son of Andrew and Martha Wilson Weldon, died in 1854, aged 18 years.

⁴ Emma J., youngest daughter of Andrew and Martha Wilson Weldon, is not married. She resides at St. John. She gave many years of her life to the care of her aged and infirm mother, and is a much esteemed and devoted Christian lady.

The account of the family of Martha Wilson and her husband Andrew Weldon here closes.

³ Jane Ruth Wilson, fourth daughter of Benjamin and Martha Dixon Wilson, married William P. Sayre, of Dorchester, in 1828. Mr. Sayre succeeded his Father in the office of Sheriff, which office he held for many years. The family of William P. and Jane R. Wilson Sayre, consisted of three daughters and a son, named Mary, Charles J., Amelia, and Martha J. R. ³ Mrs. Sayre died in 1835, aged 29 years. Mr. Sayre died in Summerside, P. E. Island, in 1872, aged 70.

⁴ Mary, the eldest daughter of William P. and Jane R. Wilson Sayre, is not married and resides at Richibacto.

⁴ Charles J., only son of William P. and Jane R. Wilson Sayre, is a lawyer residing at Richibucto. He represented the County of Kent in the Local Parliment for some years. He married Miss Mary Marshall. They have children named William P., Frederick Smith, James Francis, Mary Louise, Edith Emily, Elizabeth Travis, and Fanny Smith, none of whom are married.

⁴ Amelia, second daughter of William P. and Jane R. Wilson Sayre, married Mr. Daniel Murray. They went to New Hampshire, where Mrs. Murray died soon after her marriage leaving no issue.

⁴ Martha J. R. youngest daughter of William P. and Jane R. Wilson Sayre, married Ichabod L. Steeves. They resided at Summerside, P. E. Island, and their children were named

Charles, Florence, Emma, Annie, William P., Harry Robinson, and Alfred A. Mrs. Steeves died in 1875, aged 39 years, and Mr. Steeves died in 1882.

[5] Charles, eldest son of Ichabod L. and Martha J. R. Sayre Steeves, is a merchant in Chicago, U. S. He married Miss Ellen McEwen, and they have children named Alfred and Helen.

[5] Florence, eldest daughter of Ichabod L. and Martha J. R. Sayre Steeves, married J. Y. Merserall. They reside at Chatham, N. B., and have children named Lulu Sayre, Winnifred, Charles and one other.

[5] Emma, second daughter of Ichabod L., and Martha J. R. Sayre Steeves, married L. S. Brown, and lives in Campbelton, N. B. This closes the account of the family of Jane Ruth Wilson and her husband, William P. Sayre.

[3] Benjamin Wilson, eldest son of Benjamin and Martha Dixon Wilson, was a mechanic. He married Miss Caroline Baker, of Barronsfield, N. S. They settled at Amherst, and had two children, named Martha and Charles Baker.

[3] Mr. Wilson died in 1881, aged 73 years. Mrs. Wilson is also deceased.

[4] Martha, only daughter of Benjamin and Caroline Baker Wilson, married Joseph Quigley, a mechanic of Amherst. They removed to Boston. Their children are named Albert and Henry; the first named, Albert, is a deaf mute. Mr. Quigley died about the year 1883. Mrs. Quigley is still living at Boston.

[4] Charles Baker, only son of Benjamin and Caroline Baker Wilson, is a farmer residing at Amherst, and is not married.

The account of the family of Benjamin Wilson and his wife, Caroline Baker here closes.

³ Fanny Black Wilson, fifth daughter of Benjamin and Martha Dixon Wilson, married Rev'd Michael Pickles, a Methodist minister, in the year 1834. Mr. Pickles was a native of Keighly, Yorkshire, England, and was sent out to labor in New-Brunswick by the Missionary Committee in London in the year 1829. He came to Sackville in 1833, immediately after the death of his first wife, who was a Miss Hayward, of Sussex, N. B. Mr. Pickles was a deeply pious and devoted man, and labored effectively upon many circuits in New Brunswick and Nova Scotia, until 1863, when he became a supernumerary. The family of Rev'd Michael and Fanny B. Wilson Pickles consisted of four sons and three daughters, named Fletcher H. Wilson, Abigail Louisa, Mary E. S., James S. H., Martha Jane, Frederic M., John D., and six others who died in childhood or infancy. Mr. Pickles took up his residence after he became a supernumerary in St. John, where he resided until his visit to his native country, during which he died at Halifax, England in 1877, in the 80th year of his age. ³ Mrs. Pickles died at Hartland, N. B., in 1881, aged 71 years.

⁴ Fletcher H. Wilson, eldest son of Rev. Michael and Fanny B. Wilson Pickles, is also a Methodist minister. He married Miss Hattie Ricketson of Annapolis, N. S., and their family consists of four sons and three daughters, named Fred Harris, John, Blakeley, Fletcher W. Thorne, Fanny H. Lucetta, Hattie Anna Ricketson, Wesley Smith Kaye, and three others who died in childhood. Mr. Pickles is an earnest, diligent and efficient minister in the church of his Fathers.

⁵ Fred H., eldest son of Rev. Fletcher H. W. and Hattie Ricketson Pickles, is a Civil Engineer, residing at or near Minneapolis, and is not married.

⁴ Abigail Louise, eldest daughter of Rev. Michael and Fanny B. Wilson Pickles, married Josiah Barnett, of London, England. They reside at Boston, Mass., and have two daughters named Fanny Elisabeth and Edith Louise. A son named Frank Ogden died in infancy.

⁴ Mary E. S., second daughter of Rev. Michael and Fanny B. Wilson Pickles, married Charles W. Harris in 1863. Mr. Harris is a farmer. They resided at Tobique, N. B. Their children were named Mary Edith, Fannie Starr, Henry Laird Pickles, William Edgar, Susan Inglis, Minnie Louisa, Charles Rupert and Hattie Louisa. Mrs. Harris died in 1887, aged 47 years.

⁵ Mary Edith, eldest daughter of Charles W. and Mary E. S. Pickles, married a Mr. Ballou, and has three children.

⁴ James S. H., second son of Rev. Michael and Fanny B. Wilson Pickles, went to England when a young man, where he married Miss Emma Brenton. He died in 1879, aged 37 years. His widow and two children, named Fanny Ruth and Florence Louise, survive.

⁴ Martha Jane, youngest daughter of Rev. Michael and Fanny B. Wilson Pickles, married William Tweedale, merchant. They resided in St. John, and their children were named Frank DeWolf, Edith May, Fred and Maud. Mrs. Tweedale died in 1884, aged 40 years. Mr. Tweedale is again married and resides at Lynn, Mass.

⁴ Frederic M., third son of Rev. Michael and Fanny B. Wilson Pickles, is a minister of the Methodist Episcopal Church, and resides in Washington State. He married Miss Mamie Maynard, and they have children named Grace Irene and Bessie.

[4] John D., youngest son of Rev. Michael and Fanny B. Wilson Pickles, is also a minister of the Methodist Episcopal Church, and resides at Worcester, Mass. He married Miss Elizabeth Seavey, of Booth Bay, Maine. They have one child named Helen Winchell. Mr. Pickles is a studious scholarly man wearing the Degree of Ph D., and an eloquent and devoted minister of his church.

This ends the account of the family of Fanny B. Wilson and her husband Rev. M. Pickles.

[3] Louisa Ann Wilson, sixth daughter of Benjamin and Martha Dixon Wilson, married Mr. James Harris in 1836. Mr. Harris was a merchant and manufacturer, residing at Portland, N. B. They had a family consisting of seven daughters and a son, named Julia E., Augusta J., Louisa E., Clara Charlotte, Annie Gertrude, James Stanley, Calista C. H., Laura Pauline, and another who died in infancy. Mr. Harris was the leading member of one of the first and largest Iron manufacturing firms in the Provinces. He was an indefatigable worker, and a pious and much esteemed Christian gentleman. [3] Mrs. Harris was a universally beloved and esteemed Lady. She died in 1887, aged 74 years, and Mr. Harris died in 1888, aged 84 years.

[4] Julia E., eldest daughter of James and Louisa A. Wilson Harris, married Mr. William Esson of Halifax. They resided at Halifax, where Mr. Esson was engaged in the West India trade. Their family consists of four sons and a daughter, named John S., William B., Frank G., Arthur Campbell and Laura Pauline.

[4] Augusta J., second daughter of James and Louisa A. Wilson Harris, is not married.

⁴ Louisa E., third daughter of James and Louisa A. Wilson Harris, married Amos S. Wilson, a lawyer, residing at Dorchester, a son of the late Richard Wilson of Sackville. They had one daughter named Annie Louise. Mr. Wilson died in 1869 about two years after his marriage. Mrs. Wilson resides at St. John.

⁵ Annie Louise, only daughter of Amos S. and Louisa E. Harris Wilson, died in 1885, aged 14 years.

⁴ Clara Charlotte, fourth daughter of James and Louisa Ann Wilson Harris, married Charles Romans, a merchant of Halifax, N. S. They have children named James Stanley, Charles, Mabel, and Myra. One other died in infancy.

⁴ Annie Gertrude, fifth daughter of James and Louisa Ann Wilson Harris, married John Thornton of Montreal. They reside at St. John, where Mr. Thornton was engaged in the business with Mr. Harris. They have children named Stanley H., Nora, Paul, Arthur, Helen, and John.

⁴ James Stanley, only son of James S. and Louisa Ann Wilson Harris, died unmarried, aged 22 years.

⁴ Calista C. H., sixth daughter of James and Louisa Ann Wilson Harris, married Mr. James Robertson, who was for some years associated with Mr. Harris in the business, and is now manager thereof. They have children named Edith, Harold, and Kathleen. One other died in infancy.

⁴ Laura Pauline, youngest daughter of James and Louisa Ann Wilson Harris, married Mr. James Mowatt, Banker. They reside at Moncton, and have two children, named Margery Louise and Frances Calista. This closes the account of the family of Louisa Ann Wilson and her husband James Harris.

3 Charles Wilson, second son of Benjamin and Martha Dixon Wilson, married Miss Margaret Merry, of Chatham, N. B., in the year 1838. They resided for a time at Chatham and then removed to St. John, and Mr. Wilson entered the employ of his brother-in-law, Mr. Harris, in which he remained for many years. The family of Charles and Margaret Merry Wilson consisted of four daughters and two sons, named Louisa, Archie, Emma, Martha, Frederic C., Florence, and two others who died in infancy. 3 Mr. Charles Wilson died in 1889, aged 74 years. Mrs. Wilson is still living.

4 Louisa, eldest daughter of Charles and Margaret Merry Wilson, died unmarried in 1858, aged 19 years.

4 Archie, eldest son of Charles and Margaret Merry Wilson, married a Miss Morrison. He was a Telegraph Operator and resided at St. John. They had a family of four sons named as follows: Normack Royal, John Morrison, Charles Archibald and James Harris. 4 Mr. Wilson died in 1884, aged 43 years. His widow still lives at St. John.

4 Emma, second daughter of Charles and Margaret Merry Wilson, married Alfred Roop, of Clementsport, N. S. They had two children who died in childhood. Mrs. Roop also died in 1878, aged 36 years.

4 Martha, third daughter of Charles and Margaret Merry Wilson, married Henry Ballentine. They reside in Boston, Mass., and their children are named Arnold A. and Arthur Charles. One other died in childhood.

4 Fred C., second son of Charles and Margaret Merry Wilson, resides in New York. He married Miss Ella Abbington. They have six children named Charles F., Florence Mabel, Harry, Emily M., Ella, and another.

[4] Florence, youngest daughter of Charles and Margaret Merry Wilson, died unmarried, aged 23 years.

This closes the account of the family of Charles and Margaret Wilson.

[3] Hannah Caroline Wilson, youngest daughter of Benjamin and Martha Dixon Wilson, married James Potter, of Clementsport, N. S., in 1852. Mr. Potter was a farmer and was also engaged in milling. He died in 1888, aged 86 years. Mrs. Potter is still living and residing in St. John. They had no family.

The posterity of Martha Dixon and her husband Benjamin Wilson is as follows:

	Born.	Living.	Dead.
Children	12	1	11
Grand Children	52	24	28
Great Grand Children	130	106	24
Great Great Grand Children	43	39	4
	237	170	67

GENEALOGY OF EDWARD DIXON AND HIS WIFE MARY SMITH.

CHAPTER VIII.

[2] EDWARD, second son of Charles and Susannah Coates Dixon, resided at Sackville on the homestead farm of his Father. He married Mary Smith, daughter of John Smith, who was a Yorkshire Methodist Local Preacher and lived for a time at Falmouth, N. S., where several of his family (including Mary above named) were baptised by the Rev. Freeborn Garretson. Mr. Smith removed from Falmouth and settled at Parrsboro, where a number of his descendants still remain. His wife was a sister of Thomas Bowser, one of the early Yorkshire settlers of Sackville.

The family of Edward and Mary Smith Dixon, who were married in 1802, bore the following names:

Charles,	Born 1803.	Edwin,	Born 1805.
Elisabeth,	" 1806.	Jane Bamford,	" 1808.
John Edward,	" 1811.	George Smith, } twins,	1814.
Rufus Smith,	" 1816.	William Coates }	
James Dunbar,	" 1819.		

Another, born in 1810, died in infancy.

Mr. Dixon followed farming with fair success for a number of years. In 1825 he entered into an arrangement with a Mr. Venning to build a ship for the English market. The arrangement was carried into effect the year following. In the mean time the price of ships had fallen off so greatly that the enterprise resulted in heavy financial loss. After this, Mr. Dixon confined his attention to his farm until 1842, when he rented his farm and devoted the greater part of his time to visiting remote and sparsely settled portions of the surrounding country, assisting in holding religious services, distributing books of a religious character, and striving to promote the spiritual welfare of the people. This work he continued until near the close of his life. Mr. Dixon was for over half a century a zealous and consistent member of the Methodist Church, a large portion of which period he held the offices of Trustee, Steward and Leader, in all of which he diligently and faithfully labored to promote the advancement of God's cause. Mrs. Dixon was also a deeply pious and devoted member of the same church for an equal period of time. She died in the year 1854, aged 74 years. Mr. Dixon survived his wife about seven years and died in 1861, aged 85 years, nearly.

3 Charles, eldest son of Edward and Mary Smith Dixon, when a young man evinced a decided prediliction for a mechanical occupation in preference to farming, and chose a carpenter's trade, in which, without serving any apprenticeship, he became a proficient in a short time. He married Miss Sarah Boultenhouse in the year 1827. Shortly after his marriage he removed to Windsor, N. S., where he followed his occupation until 1831, when he returned to Sackville where he resided the remainder of his life. He was an excellent mechanic and was both architect and builder of many of the best buildings erected in Sackville during his time. In 1850 he engaged in ship building, which he followed about seven years, which

did not prove a financial success. He was an active and prominent man in the community, a leading magistrate, a zealous promoter of the cause of temperance, and filled the positions of Trustee, Leader and Local Preacher in the Methodist Church, of which both he and Mrs. Dixon were lifelong and devoted members. Mr. Dixon died in the year 1864, in the 61st year of his age. Mrs. Dixon died in the year 1884, aged 74 years. The family of Charles and Sarah Boultenhouse Dixon, consisted of Charles, who died at the age of 11 years, Sarah, Mary Elisabeth, John E., William B., Christopher E., Charlotte J., Robert Y., Charles, Henry Arthur, and Frederic Allison who died in childhood.

4 Sarah, eldest daughter of Charles and Sarah Boultenhouse Dixon, married Edward Cogswell, Esq., of Sackville, whose first wife was Miss Ruth Crane as stated in Chapter VI. They reside at Sackville and have no family. Mr. Cogswell is one of the highly respected citizens of Sackville and is interested in an Iron Foundry.

4 Mary Elizabeth, second daughter of Charles and Sarah Boultenhouse Dixon, married Thomas Pickard in 1854. They reside at Sackville, where Mr. Pickard for many years held the Professorship of Mathematics in the Mount Allison Academy and College. When he retired from that position he engaged in farming. In 1874 he was elected one of the representatives of Westmoreland County, in the local Parliment, and served the usual quadrennial term. The family of Thomas and Mary E. Dixon Pickard consisted of one daughter and three sons, named Sarah Burpee, Humphrey F., Charles A., Thomas E. Dwight, and two others named Mary Alice and Edward Dwight, who died in childhood.

GENEALOGY OF EDWARD DIXON.

⁵ Sarah Burpee, eldest daughter of Thomas and Mary E. Dixon Pickard, is not married and resides with her parents.

⁵ Humphrey F., eldest son of Thomas and Mary E. Dixon Pickard, is not married, and is engaged in merchandise at Sackville.

⁵ Charles A., second son of Thomas and Mary E. Dixon Pickard, is a leading merchant of Sackville. He married Miss Margaret L. Stockton, of Sussex, N. B. They have an infant child named Kenneth Stockton.

⁵ Thomas E. Dwight, youngest son of Thomas and Mary E. Dixon Pickard is not married, and assists his brother in the store.

⁴ John Edward, eldest son of Charles and Sarah Boultenhouse Dixon, when about sixteen years of age went to California, where he was engaged in mining operations and resided at San Francisco. He was never married. His death occurred recently, aged 57 years.

⁴ William Bedford, second son of Charles and Sarah Boultenhouse Dixon, married Miss Maria Hallet, of Kings county, N. B., who died in 1875, leaving an infant child, who also died in infancy. Mr. Dixon married a widow lady, Mrs. Edward B. Dixon, for his second wife. They have no family. Mr. Dixon is engaged in the Iron Foundry business with Mr. Cogswell and others.

⁴ Christopher E., third son of Charles and Sarah Boultenhouse Dixon, in early life went to sea and became a Shipmaster, which he followed for a time, and then engaged in the Ship Broker business at Greenock, Scotland, and afterward at Antwerp. He now resides in London, England. He married Miss

Mary E. Foster, of Yorkshire, England. They have two children named Florence May, and Edwin George.

⁴ Charlotte J., third daughter of Charles and Sarah Boultenhouse Dixon, married Rev. Thomas D. Hart, Methodist minister, in 1864, and they have a family named, Charlotte Elizabeth, Joseph A. F., Sarah L., Louisa H., Mary L. E., Edward R. K., Alice Maria, Frederick W., Lillian M. D., Cecilia May, and one other named Emmeline, who died in infancy. Rev. Mr. Hart has been thirty years in the ministry, and occupied many circuits in Prince Edwards Island and Nova Scotia, with great acceptance, and is still an earnest and faithful laborer in his Master's Vineyard.

⁵ Charlotte Elizabeth, eldest daughter of Rev. Thomas D. and Charlotte J. Dixon Hart, is an educated young lady, and is employed as a teacher in one of the Methodist Mission Schools in Japan.

⁵ Joseph A. F., eldest son of Rev. Thomas D. and Charlotte J. Dixon Hart, is preparing for the ministry.

⁵ Sarah L., second daughter of Rev. Thomas D. and Charlotte J. Dixon Hart, is a teacher in a Methodist Mission School at Chilliwack, British Columbia. None of the family of Rev. Thomas D. Charlotte J. Dixon Hart are married.

⁴ Robert Y., fifth son of Charles and Sarah Boultenhouse Dixon, also chose a sea faring life, and is a successful ship master. He married Miss Hannah Chubbuck in 1872. Their home is principally on shipboard. They have a son named Charles. Two others died in infancy.

⁴ Charles, sixth son of Charles and Sarah Boultenhouse Dixon, also chose a seafaring life, and was advancing in his profession, when the ship in which he sailed as first Officer, was

lost, with all on board, in the year 1867. He was in the 23d year of his age.

⁴ Henry Arthur, seventh son of Charles and Sarah Boultenhouse Dixon, also went to sea in a ship of which his brother Christopher E. was master. He died of Cholera on board the ship in the year 1866, aged 19 years, and was buried at sea.

The account of the family of Charles Dixon and Sarah Boultenhouse is here closed.

³ Edwin, the second son of Edward and Mary Smith Dixon, married Martha, second daughter of Thomas Anderson, of Coles Island, in the year 1827. They settled at Sackville, and their children were named George Smith, Mary Ann, Martha Jane, Jerusha, Thomas Edward, William Coates, Ruth, John, Charles and Elizabeth. Mrs. Dixon died in the year 1855, aged 45 years. Mr. Dixon married a second wife in 1856— Miss Jerusha, daughter of Mr. John Anderson, a niece of his former wife. They had children named Archdale, Claudine, Hiawatha, Adraina and Edwin Clay. Mr. Dixon was an upright, God-fearing and much respected man. He was not a member of any church, though he was a frequent attendant upon the services of the Baptist Church, of which both of his wives were members. His death occurred in July, 1887, when within a few days of completing his 82d year, and resulted from a fall from a loaded wagon. which inflicted injuries that proved fatal. His widow still survives.

George Smith, eldest son of Edwin and Martha Anderson Dixon, married Esther, daughter of Frederic Sears. They resided at Sackville where Mr. Dixon followed farming and milling. Their family consisted of five sons and one daughter, named Frank, Martha, Chipman, William Coates, Edward

AND HIS WIFE, MARY SMITH.

Bowes John, and two who died in infancy. Mrs. Dixon died in 1884. Mr. Dixon still survives.

⁵ Frank, eldest son of George S. and Esther Sears Dixon, married Miss Mary Ayr, and resides at Moncton, where he is in the employ of the Government Railway. They have children named George and Charles. Two others died in infancy.

⁵ Martha, only daughter of George and Esther Sears Dixon, married John Fenton. They resided at Sackville and had children named John and Leonora. Two others died in infancy.

⁵ Chipman, second son of George and Esther Sears Dixon, married Miss Lucy Wry. They reside at Moncton, where Mr. Dixon is employed on the Government Railway. They have a child named Bessie.

⁵ William Coates, third son of George and Esther Sears Dixon, is farming at Ladners Landing, British Columbia, and is not married.

⁵ Edward Bowes, fourth son of George S. and Esther Sears Dixon, is in Norwich, Connecticut. He married Miss Rose Malcoln, of that town.

⁵ John, youngest son of George and Esther Sears Dixon, is not married, and is at Moncton in the employ of the Government Railway.

⁴ Mary Ann, eldest daughter of Edwin and Martha Anderson Dixon, married James Anderson, son of John Anderson, late of Sackville. They reside at Upper Dorchester. They have children named George, Edwin Clay, Carrie Clifford, Martin Luther, Warren Cutter, and Daisy Ruth. Mr. Anderson owns a valuable farm which he has reclaimed from the wilderness,

and also, an esteblishment of Mills, and manufactures lumber of various kinds extensively.

⁵ George, the eldest son of James and Mary A. Dixon Anderson, is not married and resides with his Father.

⁵ Edwin Clay, second son of James and Mary A. Dixon Anderson, resides in St. John where he occupies a position in the Electric Light Works of that city.

⁵ Carrie Clifford, eldest daughter of James and Mary A. Dixon Anderson, married William Venning Black, a farmer and only son of the late Martin Black, of Dorchester. They reside in Dorchester and have children named Ralph Morris and Meta Louisa.

⁵ Martin Luther, third son of James and Mary A. Dixon Anderson, married Miss Alice Weldon, daughter of Amos Weldon, Esq., of Dorchester. They have one child and reside at Amherst, where Mr. Anderson is engaged in merchandise.

⁵ Warren Cutter, fourth son of James and Mary A. Dixon Anderson, married Miss Annie Scurr, of Sackville, as stated on page 111. They reside at Dorchester, where Mr. Dixon is engaged in farming and lumbering with his Father.

⁵ Daisy Ruth, youngest daughter of James and Mary A. Dixon Anderson, is not married.

⁴ Martha Jane, second daughter of Edwin and Martha Anderson Dixon, married Amos Tingley, a farmer of Sackville. They had children named Emma, Heber, Harvey, Edwin, Lee, and Mary, and four others who died in infancy.

⁵ Emma, eldest daughter of Amos and Martha Jane Dixon Tingley, married a Mr. Cleveland, of Amherst, where they resided. They had no family and Mrs. Cleveland died early.

⁵ Heber, eldest son of Amos and Martha Jane Dixon Ting-

ley, married Miss McGinness. They reside at Sackville and have two children.

⁵ Harvey, second son of Amos and Martha J. Dixon Tingley, is not married and follows seafaring.

⁵ Edwin, third son of Amos and Martha J. Dixon Tingley, is not married and resides at Dorchester with his mother.

⁵ Lee, fourth son of Amos and Martha J. Dixon Tingley, lives in Boston, Mass. Not married.

⁵ Mary, second daughter of Amos and Martha J. Dixon Tingley, married Frank Watson. They live in Boston, Mass., and have a child named Alta Pearl. Mr. and Mrs. Amos Tingley are still living, but have lived separately for many years.

⁴ Jerusha, third daughter of Edwin and Martha Anderson Dixon, married Stuart Estabrooks, a farmer, of Sackville. They had one daughter named Mary, and two children who died in infancy, and two others who died in early life. ⁴ Mrs. Estabrooks died many years since, and Mr. Estabrooks is again married.

⁵ Mary, the daughter above mentioned, is not married, and resides at home with her father.

⁴ Thomas Edward, second son of Edwin and Martha Anderson Dixon, died in the 18th year of his age from injuries he received by falling from a load of fire wood, which passed over him.

₄ William Coates, third son of Edwin and Martha Anderson Dixon, went to Australia when about eighteen years of age, and resides at Ballarat East, and follows mining. He is married and has children named Amy, Alice, Edwin, Charles, Lucy, Alfred, James, George and Bertie.

⁴ Ruth, fourth daughter of Edwin and Martha Anderson

Dixon, married George A. Hardy, a farmer of Andover, Mass. They have children named Eva Adelaide, and Henry George. Two others Edwin Dixon and Edgar died in infancy.

₄ John, fourth son of Edwin and Martha Anderson Dixon, married Miss Alice Ann Atherton, of Lowell, Mass. They reside in Pennsylvania, and have children named Elizabeth Atherton, Charles Edwin, and Arthur Anderson, all unmarried.

₄ Charles, fifth son of Edwin and Martha Dixon, followed the sea and became a shipmaster. He married Charity Elizabeth Dixon, and they had a daughter named Winnifred Tempest, as stated on page 67. Mr. Dixon died suddenly of heart disease while in the act of getting his vessel under weigh, when about to leave port.

₄ Elizabeth, youngest daughter of Edwin and Martha Anderson Dixon, is not married and resides with her sister at Andover, Mass.

₄ Archdale, eldest son of Edwin and Jerusha Anderson Dixon, married Miss Rachel Cole, and resides at Aboushaggan, and is engaged in farming and milling. Their first child died in infancy. Mrs. Dixon died in 1890 leaving an infant a few days old.

₄ Claudine, eldest daughter of Edwin and Jerusha Anderson Dixon, married Charles Ayr. They reside in Albert county, N. B. and have two children, Mabel and Maud.

₄ Hiawatha, second son of Edwin and Jerusha Anderson Dixon, is recently married to a Miss Copp, and resides at Aboushaggan, and is engaged in milling.

₄ Adraina, second daughter of Edwin Jerusha Anderson Dixon, is not married and resides at Lowell, Mass.

AND HIS WIFE, MARY SMITH.

⁴ Edwin Clay, youngest son of Edwin and Jerusha Anderson Dixon, is not married and resides with his mother at Aboushaggan. The account of the family of Edwin Dixon here closes.

³ Elizabeth, eldest daughter of Edward and Mary Smith Dixon, married James Chubbuck in the year 1827. Mr. Chubbuck was a master mechanic, of Maine, U. S., and was employed by Mr. Dixon and Mr. Venning to superintend the building of a ship for them in 1826. After their marriage Mr. and Mrs. Chubbuck removed to Windsor, N. S., where they resided about twenty years, and then removed to Parrsboro, where Mr. C. followed his occupation until his death in the year 1856. After the death of Mr. C., Mrs. Chubbuck removed with a portion of the family to Sackville, where she died in the year 1859, aged 53 years. The family of James and Elizabeth Dixon Chubbuck, consisted of Mary Elizabeth, Sarah A., Amelia J., Hannah Augusta, Charles E. D., and six others who died in infancy.

⁴ Mary Elisabeth, eldest daughter of James and Elisabeth Dixon Chubbuck, married Alexander P. Bradley, a merchant of Parrsboro, where they resided for some years. They now reside at Ottawa, where Mr. Bradley is Secretary of the Department of Railways and Canals. The family of Alexander P. and Mary E. Chubbuck Bradley consists of Annie R., William Inglis, and Sarah. Two others died infancy.

⁵ Annie R., eldest daughter of Alexander P. and Mary E. Chubbuck Bradley, married Alfred G. Kingston, of the Public Works Department, Ottawa, and they have children named Margaret Clare, Laurence B., John and Sarah (twins), and Anna Bradley

⁵ William Inglis, only son of Alexander P. and Mary E. Chubbuck Bradley, is a medical man and not married.

⁵ Sarah, second daugnter of Alexander P. and Mary E. Chubbuck Bradley, died in 1875, aged sixteen years.

⁴ Sarah A., second daughter of James and Elizabeth Dixon Chubbuck, is not married, and resides with her brother at Ottawa.

⁴ Amelia J., third daughter of James and Elizabeth Dixon Chubbuck, is also unmarried, and resides with her sister, Mrs. Bradley.

⁴ Hannah A., fourth daughter of James and Elizabeth Dixon Chubbuck, is married to Robert Y. Dixon, ship master, as previously stated in this chapter.

⁴ Charles E. D., only son of James and Elizabeth Dixon Chubbuck, holds a position in the Department of Inland Revenue, at Ottawa. He married Miss Harriet Burrows, and they had children named Leonard B., Charles Inglis, and Harriet F. Mrs. Chubbuck died in 1885. Mr. Chubbuck married Miss May Newsome for his second wife. They have an infant daughter named Madge Rainsford.

This closes the account of Elizabeth Dixon and James Chubbuck's family.

³ Jane Bamford, second daughter of Edward and Mary Smith Dixon, married David Lyons in January 1830. David Lyons was a shipmaster and also a mechanic. He followed coasting a number of years and then sailed on foreign voyages. They resided at Sackville, and their children were named Rufus Dixon, Annie M., David, William Henry, and Mary Ann, two of whom, ⁴ Annie M. and ⁴ David, died in childhood. Capt. David Lyons died at Benin, on the coast of Africa, of

fever, on the 22d of October, 1865, aged 57 years, and Mrs. Jane B. Lyons died at Sackville January 1st, 1881, aged 72 years.

4 Rufus D., eldest son of Capt. David and Jane B. Dixon Lyons, was also a shipmaster and excelled in his profession. He married Miss Emily Miles, of London, England, in 1855. They had one daughter named Emily. Mrs. Lyons died in 1865, aged 32 years. Capt. R. D. Lyons married for a second wife Miss Janet Thomson, of Liverpool, in 1870. They had two children named Rufus and Henry. Capt. Lyons died at Iquique in the year 1873. After her husband's death, Mrs. Lyons removed with her family to Beechworth, Victoria, Australia, where she died in September, 1885. Her son Rufus died in childhood.

5 Emily, only daughter of Capt. Rufus D. and Emily Miles Lyons, married Herbert Jackson, a farmer, of Victoria, Australia, and they have three children.

5 Henry, youngest son of Capt. Rufus and Janet Thomson Lyons, is not married.

4 William Henry, youngest son of Captain David and Jane B. Dixon Lyons, is also a shipmaster standing high in his profession, and has for many years been in command of large steamships plying between European and South American ports. He married Miss Mary Thomson, of Liverpool, in 1873. Their home is in England. They have children named Jane, Henry, William Rufus, Richard Sackville, Mary Edith, George Herbert, Ernest Thomson and Howard Maitland, one of whom (Richard Sackville) died in infancy.

4 Mary Ann, youngest daughter of Captain David and Jane B. Dixon Lyons, was never married. She acquired an

education and obtained a first-class Teachers' license and taught school twenty years at Sackville. She was a successful teacher and an earnest and zealous christian worker. She was stricken down with paralysis while engaged in conducting a "Band of Hope" meeting in August, 1885. She lingered until 1887, when she died at the age of 46 years.

The account of the family of Jane B. Dixon and her husband David Lyons here closes.

3 John E., third son of Edward and Mary Smith Dixon, left the home of his youth in the spring of 1833, to seek his fortune in the United States, and settled in Ohio where he remained several years. He turned his attention to mechanical pursuits and soon became an excellent carpenter and builder. He married Miss Thirza Dille, of Euclid, Ohio. They had two daughters named Amelia C. and Evangelia, and two sons named Edward and John-Forrest, who died in childhood. Mrs. Dixon died in 1849, aged 32 years. In 1850 Mr. Dixon married Miss Mary Ann Wolf. They had one daughter named Mary who died in childhood. They resided at Marine City and also at Detroit, where Mr. Dixon was engaged in ship building. The ship building business proving unprofitable, Mr. Dixon removed with his family to the country in 1860 and applied himself to farming. In 1864 he was employed to go to Alabama to work at the finishing of some gunboats for the United States Government, and soon after was taken ill and died on the 19th of June of that year, aged 52 years. Within a few years after his arrival in Ohio he became a member of the "Disciples of Christ," and occasionally exercised his talents in preaching and holding meetings in connection with

that people. His widow survived him many years and died in the year 1887, aged 78 years.

[4] Amelia C., eldest daughter of John E. and Thirza Dille Dixon, married Andrew Little, in September, 1865. They resided at Ionia, Michigan, and their children were named Mary Catherine, Flora Evangelia, James Edward, Lora Dixon and Forest Andrew. The two first named died in childhood, and [5] Lora, the third named, died in 1890, aged 19 years. Mrs. Little died in 1875, aged 33 years. Mr. Little and his two sons still survive.

[4] Evangelia, second daughter of John E. and Thirza Dille Dixon, married Ambrose Smith, farmer, in the year 1869. They reside at Woods Corners, Ionia, Michigan, and have one son and four daughters, named Herbert Lee, Bertha Lucile, Mabel Claire, Carrie May, and Lucetta Amelia.

[5] Bertha Lucile, eldest daughter of Ambrose and Evangelia Dixon Smith, married Rosalvo A. Grover in 1889. They reside at Woodward Lake, Michigan, and have a daughter named Mildred Evangelia. Mr. Grover is an Engineer, but at present engaged in farming.

The account of the family of John E. Dixon here closes.

[3] George Smith, fourth son of Edward and Mary Smith Dixon; was accidentally killed by being thrown from a horse. The sad event occurred in August 1824 in the eleventh year of his age.

[3] William Coates, twin brother of George Smith, served an apprenticeship with his brother-in-law, James Chubbuck, at Windsor, Nova Scotia. When his apprenticeship closed he returned to Sackville, where he followed his occupation some years. In the year 1841 he married Miss Mary

J. Trueman, third daughter of Thomas Trueman, of Point DeBute. They resided at Sackville until the death of Mrs. Dixon in 1844, who left no issue. Shortly after the death of his wife, Mr. Dixon visited his brother, John E., at Detroit, Michigan, and subsequently became associated with him in ship-building. In 1848 he married Miss Harriet E. Arnold, a native of London, England. They resided at Detroit and Marine City until 1865, when they removed to and settled on a farm at Maidstone, Essex County, Ontario. Mrs. Dixon's parents and their family had previously settled in the same vicinity. The family of William C. and Harriet E. Arnold Dixon consisted of six sons and five daughters, named George, Harriet-Emma, Mary Jane, Susan, Helen, Charles, William Edwin, Orville Dewey, Eunice Emily, Henry James, and James Rufus, two of whom, George and Orville Dewey, died in childhood and infancy. Mr. Dixon is still active and vigorous, capable of much physical exertion; and has an excellent memory, is a diligent reader, with a decided preference for poetical works, and even employs some of his leisure hours in writing poetic effusions, a talent which only developed itself when its possessor had nearly reached his three score years and ten.

[4] Harriet Emma, eldest daughter of William C. and Harriet Arnold Dixon, married George Little in 1868. Mr. Little is a farmer, residing near Maidstone. They have children named Charles William, Susan Felicia, Harriet Emma, Arthur Wesley, Mary Jane, George Alfred, Helen Louise, Cora May, Roy Dixon, Frederic and a babe.

[4] Mary Jane, second daughter of William C. and Harriet E. Arnold Dixon, married Samuel James in 1871. They reside in

Michigan and follow farming. Their family consists of four children, named William, Clara Elinor, Nellie, and George Herbert, who died in childhood.

4 Susan, third daughter of William C. and Harriet E. Arnold Dixon, married Thomas Rush, a native of England. Mr. Rush is Postmaster at Essex Centre, where he resides. The family of Thomas and Susan Dixon Rush consists of Walter Leigh, Harriet, Thomas Dixon, Bernice Ellen, John Edward, Frank Boughton, Mildred Eva, and Elsie Irene. Two of the above named, Walter Leigh and Frank Boughton. died in childhood.

4 Helen, fourth daughter of William C. and Harriet E. Arnold Dixon, married David Ure, farmer, in 1878. They reside at Hurst Settlement, near Maidstone. They have children named William Dixon, Charles Wesley, Eunice Emily, Florence Myrtle, Mary Jane, and Hattie.

4 Charles, eldest surviving son of William C. and Harriet E. Arnold Dixon, married Miss Mary Elizabeth Wright, in 1880. Mr. Dixon is a mechanic and now resides at Salt Lake City, Utah. Their children are named Thomas William, Mary Ann, John, Elizabeth Maud, and another named Ethel Viola, who died in childhood.

4 William Edwin, second son of William C. and Harriet E. Arnold Dixon, married Miss Catharine Wright in 1882. They reside at Maidstone and follow farming, and have children named Henry Warren and Florence.

4 Eunice Emily, fifth daughter of William C. and Harriet E. Arnold Dixon, is a lover of music, and devotes herself to its study, practice and teaching. She resides at Essex Centre with her sister. She married James C. Connelly in 1886, and

they have a son named Edwin Dixon. Mr. Connelly has been for some time past in Oregon.

4 Henry James, third son of William C. and Harriet E. Arnold Dixon, is a watchmaker, and followed that business a number of years at Essex Centre, and afterwards in Montana. He is not married.

5 James Rufus, youngest son of William C. and Harriet E. Arnold Dixon, is not married and resides at home with his parents. This closes the account of the family of William C. Dixon and his wife Harriet Arnold.

3 Rufus Smith, sixth son of Edward and Mary Smith Dixon, when young, learned, and for a time followed the shoemaking business. About the year 1842 he became strongly impressed with the conviction that he was called to the ministry. He exercised his gifts as a local preacher for several years and in 1848 joined the East Maine M. E. Conference. In 1849 he married Miss Mary A. Burnham, daughter of William Burnham, formerly of Sackville, N. B. They had children named Frances E. and William R., and one who died in infancy. Mrs. Dixon died of consumption in 1859. In 1862 Mr. Dixon married Miss Emily Baker, a teacher. They had children named James Albert, Effie E, Grace May, and Daisy Ethel. Of the foregoing, 4 James Albert died in 1876, aged 13 years, and 4 Effie E., died in infancy. Mrs. Dixon died suddenly in the year 1887. Mr. Dixon still survives, and resides at Montville, Me. He has for several years sustained a supernumerary relation, but still preaches occasionally.

4 Frances E., eldest daughter of Rev. Rufus S. and Mary A. Burnham Dixon, married John Cary in 1877. They reside at Montville. Me., where Mr. Cary is engaged in agricultural

and mercantile pursuits. They have two sons named Daniel E. and James Dixon.

⁴ William R., only son of Rev. Rufus and Mary A. Burnham Dixon, when a young man, went to South Dakota and engaged in stock raising. He married Miss Alma Loomis. They had a son named Charles William and a babe. Mr. Dixon died in 1888, aged 32 years.

⁴ Grace May and ⁴ Daisy Ethel, surviving daughters of Rev. Rufus S. and Emily Baker Dixon, are not married, and reside with their Father at Montville.

The account of the family of Rev. Rufus Dixon here closes.

³ James D., youngest son of Edward and Mary Smith Dixon, married Miss Eunice Black, second daughter of George M. Black, of Dorchester. They occupied a part of the old Homestead farm of his Father and Grandfather. Mr. Dixon was appointed Collector of Customs in 1855 and held that office until 1882. He was also for several years connected with the Provincial Board of Agriculture, and took an active interest in agricultural affairs and was on several occasions a delegate to select stock for importation. In 1877 he retired from the farm, leaving it in the hands of his sons, and erected a cottage nearer the Village on a small portion of the property of his Grandfather, where he still resides. The family of James D. and Eunice Black Dixon consisted of Mary Emily, Samuel Edgar, Alfred Black, Clementina Clara, Frederic Agtha, and Louise Cardy.

⁴ Mary Emily, eldest daughter of James D. and Eunice Black Dixon, married Joseph Archibald in 1867. Mr. Archibald was a native of Truro, N. S., and was then in charge of the office of the Western Union Telegraph Office at Sackville.

After residing at Sackville a few years they removed to St. John, and soon after Mr. Archibald's health failed and he was compelled to give up business and return to Sackville. Mr. Archibald died in 1876. The family of Joseph and Mary E. Dixon Archibald consisted of Frederic A., Herbert Dixon, and Frank Heustis who died in infancy. In 1878 Mrs. Archibald was married to Harmon Humphrey, who owned a large farm in Sackville. They had one daughter named Ella Clementina, who died in 1886, aged five years. Mr. Humphrey died suddenly in July 1887, aged 56 years. Mrs. Humphrey resides with her parents at Sackville.

[5] Frederic A., eldest son of Joseph and Mary E. Dixon Archibald, is not married, and is now in a drug store at Salt Lake City.

[5] Herbert Dixon, second son of Joseph and Mary E. Dixon Archibald, is a telegraph operator, and has charge of the Canada Pacific Telegraph Office at Sackville.

[4] Samuel Edgar, eldest son of James and Eunice Black Dixon, is a farmer residing at Sackville. He married Miss Emma Carter, daughter of Joseph Carter of Point De Bute, in 1870. They have a family of three sons, named Walter Irving, James Leaman and Clarence Edgar.

[4] Alfred Black, second son of James D. and Eunice Black Dixon, married Miss Florence Freeman in 1878, youngest daughter of Samuel Freeman of Amherst. They resided in Sackville, and followed farming, and have children named Leonard Freeman, Ernest, Clementina, and Herbert Jackson. Mr. Dixon and family have recently removed to British Columbia.

AND HIS WIFE, MARY SMITH.

₄ Clementina C., second daughter of James D. and Eunice Black Dixon, died in 1875, aged twenty years.

₄ Frederic Agtha, youngest son of James D. and Eunice Black Dixon, is a graduate of Mount Allison College. He married Miss Maggie J Patterson, daughter of James Patterson, of Sackville. They have no family except an adopted child named Gladys. Mr. Dixon is farming on a portion of the old homestead of his ancestors.

₄ Louise Cardy, youngest daughter of James D. and Eunice Black Dixon, married Rev. William Arthur Black, (eldest son of Rev. A. B. Black, of Amherst, N. S.,) in the year 1881. Mr. Black is a graduate of Mount Allison College, and a Minister and Presiding Elder in the Northwest Iowa Conference of the M. E. Church, and resides at Algona. They have one daughter named Ella Louise, another named Emma died in infancy.

This closes the account of the family of James Dixon and Eunice Black.

The posterity of Edward Dixon and Mary Smith is as follows:

	Born.	Living.	Dead.
Children	10	3	7
Grand Children	62	40	22
Great Grand Children	147	120	27
Great Great Grand Children	23	19	4
Totals,	242	˙182	60

GENEALOGY OF WILLIAN COATES DIXON AND HIS WIFE MATILDA BECKWITH.

CHAPTER IX.

[2]WILLIAM COATES, youngest son of Charles and Susannah Coates Dixon, after attaining his majority, continued to assist his Father and Brother Edward in the management of the farm until the year 1808, when he entered into partnership with his brother-in-law Benjamin Wilson at Dorchester, where they conducted a mercantile business. They were also engaged in lumbering operations, and during a portion of this partnership period, Mr. Dixon resided at Shediac, where in the year 1820 he married Miss Matilda Beckwith, daughter of John Steadman Beckwith, Esq. Soon after his marriage the partnership business terminated and Mr. Dixon and family returned to Sackville and settled on his farm where they remained until the year 1827. Then they sold the farm to Mr. Crane and returned to Shediac where they kept a hotel for a few years, and then removed to, and settled upon a farm at Buctouche, where they resided until death. The family of [2] William Coates and Matilda Beckwith Dixon consisted of three sons and three daughters named as follows:

Horatio Edward, born July 25, 1821.

Mary A., born December 9, 1822.

Lavinia Caroline, born August 11, 1826.

Caroline Lavinia, born September 8, 1830.
John Steadman, born October 7, 1833.
William James, born May 27, 1836.
One of the above named (Lavinia Caroline) died in infancy.

2 Mr. Dixon, who was quite blind for several years previous, died in 1865 in the 87th year of his age. Mrs. Dixon's death occurred quite suddenly within a few days after that of her husband, at the age of 64 years. They were life-long attendants upon the services of the Methodist Church; and services were frequently held at their house, which was ever a home for the Ministers of the Gospel. As they lived, so also they died in the faith of the Gospel.

3 Horatio Edward, eldest son of William Coates and Matilda Beckwith Dixon, was in early life engaged in a variety of pursuits, including farming, piloting and seafaring. In 1853 he married Miss Charlotte Pollard, of P. E. Island. They resided at Buctouche. Mrs. Dixon died in 1855, leaving no issue. Mr. Dixon, soon after the death of his wife, went to sea and was absent on long voyages for a number of years. In 1865 he married Miss Elisabeth Grannell and settled again upon his farm at Buctouche where he still resides. They have no family.

3 Mary A., eldest daughter of William Coates and Matilda Beckwith Dixon, lived with her parents until their decease, after which, she, with her younger sister, sold out their property and removed to St. Stephen, N. B., where she died in 1872, aged 49 years. She was not married.

3 Caroline Lavinia, youngest daughter of William Coates and Matilda Beckwith Dixon, married Mr. John Smith, a mer-

chant of Saint Stephen in the year 1870. They have no family.

[3] John Steadman, second son of William Coates and Matilda Beckwith Dixon, married Miss Elizabeth Buckerfield, daughter of an English Barrister, who came to New Brunswick about 1840, and resided for a time at Point De Bute, and finally settled on Prince Edward Island, where he died recently at an advanced age.

[3] Mr. and Mrs. Dixon reside upon a portion of the old homestead farm at Buctouche. They have children named William Henry, Cecilia Kate, Sarah Matilda, Thomas Buckerfield, Edward Algernon, Elizabeth Jane, John Steadman and Edith Sophia. None of the above named are married. The two eldest [4] William Henry, and [4] Cecilia Kate, are engaged in school teaching.

[3] William James, youngest son of William Coates and Matilda Beckwith Dixon, married Miss Jane Craig, of P. E. Island. They resided at Buctouche and had children named Walter L. and Ella. Ella died in childhood. After the death of their child, Mr. Dixon sold out and removed to St. Stephen, and subsequently to Calais, Me. Mrs. Dixon died in September 1890. Mr. Dixon still survives.

[4] Walter L., only son of William James and Jane Craig Dixon, married Miss Agnes Cochrane, and resides in Calais. They have children named William Leslie, Horatio Edward and a babe.

The account of the family of William Coates Dixon and his wife, Matilda Beckwith, here closes.

Posterity of William Coates Dixon and his wife, Matilda Beckwith:

	Born.	Living.	Dead.
Children	6	4	2
Grand Children	10	9	1
Great Grand Children	3	3	0
	19	16	3

TABLE OF POSTERITY OF CHARLES DIXON AND HIS WIFE, SUSANNAH COATES.

The following table shows the posterity of Charles Dixon and his wife Susannah Coates, and the number of each generation.

Generation.		Total.	Living.	Dead.
1st,	Charles and Susanah Dixon,	2	0	2
2d,	Children of C. and S. "	8	0	8
3d,	Grand " of C. and S. "	87	15	72
4th,	Gt. " " of C. and S. "	477	257	220
5th,	Gt. " " " of C. and S. "	1348	1039	309
6th,	Gt. " " " " of C. and S. "	849	723	126
7th,	Gt. " " " " " of C. and S. "	36	33	3
	Totals, - - - -	2807	2067	740

TABLE OF POSTERITY BY FAMILIES.

	Total.	Living.	Dead.
Charles and Susannah Dixon, - -	2	0	2
Their children, - - - - -	8	0	8
Posterity of Mary Dixon, - - -	854	645	209
" " Charles Dixon, 2d, - -	542	421	121
" " Susannah Dixon, - - -	604	433	171
" " Elizabeth Dixon, - -	172	108	64
" " Ruth Dixon, - - -	127	92	35
" " Martha Dixon, - -	237	170	67
" " Edward Dixon, - -	242	182	60
" " William Coates Dixon, -	19	16	3
Totals, - -	2807	2067	740

CONCLUDING REMARKS.

IT will be observed by all who read the foregoing pages, that the descendants of Charles and Susannah Dixon are very widely scattered. They are to be found in almost every Province of Canada and in very many of the States of the Union; in Japan, New Zealand, Australia, and some have found homes in Old England near the birthplace of their ancestors. They are also to be found filling every sphere of honest industry, and holding positions of more or less prominence in the learned professions. While a considerable portion of them have become members or adherents of other churches and religious bodies, the larger portion, it is believed, are to be found among the adherents of Methodism, the church of their ancestors. The writer recently enjoyed the unusual privilege' of being present at a family gathering in Utah, at which all the surviving generations, (five in number,) were represented. A circumstance which enables him to state that he has seen *some* of each of the *seven* generations, included in the preceding tables.

ERRATA.

PAGE.
2—Fourteenth line from top, read 1759 in place of 1795.
10—Second line from top, read preceded instead of proceeded.
24—Ninth line from top, read Buctouche instead of Butouche.
40—Sixth line from bottom, read Catherine instead of Cartharine.
42—Second line from bottom, read who instead of which.
55—Eleventh line from top, read Dixon instead of Discon.
61—Ninth line from top, read figure 3 instead of 5.
61—Fifth line from bottom, read Audy instead of Andy.
61—Fourth line from bottom, read and Arthur, once only.
81—Seventh line from, read Eaton instead of Edton.
100—Eleventh line from bottom, read Mr. instead of Wm.
102—Eighth line from bottom, read who instead of which.
107—Fourteenth line from top, read resided instead of reside.
110—Fifth line from top, omit the name "Louise."
111—Eleventh line from bottom, read Mr. instead of Wm.
112—Tenth line from top, read figure 3 instead of 5.
152—Sixth line from top, read 1793 and 1795, instead of 1898 and 1895.
169—Eighth line from bottom, read 1806 instead of 1805.

INDEX.

CONTENTS OF CHAPTER I.

	PAGES
Paper written by Charles Dixon, containing account of his early life, conversion, marriage, removal to America, etc. etc..................................	1 to 5
Author's reference to other Dixon families............	6
Mr. Dixon appointed Justice of Peace and Judge of Sessions...	7
His fellow immigrants and where they settled..........	8
His old acquaintances, and coming of John Richardson..	9
Revolutionary war breaks out ; roberry of house, etc ...	10
Coming of Refugees and Loyalists....	11
New Brunswick made a separate Province	11
Mr. Dixon a member of first Parliament.............. .	11
Members of second Parliament........................	12
Mr. Dixon appointed Collector of Customs........... ..	12
Original grantees of Sackville, and English settlers.....	13
First Methodist Church and Parsonage erected at Sackville	14
References to Mrs. Dixon and her sister and Coates family	15
Death of Mr. and Mrs. Dixon, and Family Record	16

CONTENTS OF CHAPTER II.

2 Mary Dixon marries William Chapman........	16
Copy of their family record, and their decease..........	17–18
3 William Chapman and Harriet Bent and family......	18
3 Susanna Chapman and John Greeno's family:.........	19–24
3 Elisabeth Chapman and Nehemiah Ward and family...	24–28
3 Jane Chapman and Andrew Weldon and family.... ..	28–29

3 Charles Chapman and Sarah Minard and family....... 29–31
3 Henry Chapman and Isabel Jones and family......... 31–41
3 Henry Chapman and Martha Trenholm and family..... 41
3 John Chapman and Jane Jonah and family............ 41–49
3 Richard Chapman and Jane Wells and family 49–51
3 Jennie Chapman's death............................ 51
3 Sidney Smith Chapman and Elisabeth Kay and family. 51–53
3 Mary Chapman and Luke Doyle and family... .... ·54–55
3 H. Nelson Chapman and family..................... 55
Posterity of Mary Dixon and William Chapman......... 56

CONTENTS OF CHAPTER III.

2 Charles Dixon 2d marries Rhoda Emmerson........... 57
Martha Grace marries Ebenezer Cole, the same time.... 57
2 Charles and Rhoda Dixon's family record............. 57
Death of Mrs. Rhoda Dixon........................... 58
2 Charles Dixon 2d marries Elisabeth Humphrey........ 58
Their family record................................. 58
2 Mr. Dixon and Timothy Richardson visit United States 58–59
2 Mr. Dixon's various enterprises..................... 59
His conversion to Mormonism and removal to Ohio...... 60
He starts for Salt Lake City, and meets his death....... 60–61
3 William Dixon and Elisabeth Weldon and family 61–65
3 Charles Dixon and Jane E. Metcalf and family........ 65–68
3 Hannah Dixon and John Barnes and family.......... 68–72
3 Benjamin Dixon and Mary Weldon and family......... 72–76
3 John Dixon, son of Charles and Elisabeth Humphrey... 76
3 Elisabeth Dixon and John McKinlay and family....... 76–78
3 Sidney Dixon..................................... 78
3 Leonard Dixon and Eliza Robson and family.......... 78–80
3 Jane Dixon and George H. Pepper and family......... 80–81
3 Ruth Dixon and Edward O'Hara and family.......... 82
3 Christopher F. Dixon and family.................... 82–84
3 Edward Dixon and family.......................... 84–85
3 Alfred Dixon and family........................... 85–86
3 Mary A. Dixon and Charles B. Wightman and family.. 86–88
3 Martha Dixon and Orrawell Simons and family........ 88–89
Table of posterity of Charles Dixon 2d. 90

CONTENTS OF CHAPTER IV.

2 Susanna Dixon and George Bulmer married	91
Their family record...........	92
3 Jane Bulmer and William Smith and family...........	92–95
3 Charles D. Bulmer and family	95–104
3 James B. Bulmer and family...................... ...	104–106
3 Mary Bulmer and Benjamin Scurr and family...........	106–112
3 John Bulmer and family	112–113
3 George Bulmer and family	113–115
3 Ann Bulmer and Joseph Bowser and family...........	115–116
3 Elisabeth Bulmer and Henry McLellan and family.....	116–117
3 Isabel Bulmer and James Estabrooks and family	117–120
3 Edward Bulmer and family	120–121
3 H. Nelson Bulmer and family.........	121–123
3 William Bulmer and family..........................	123–124
Posterity of Susanna Dixon and George Bulmer.........	125

CONTENTS OF CHAPTER V.

2 Elisabeth Dixon marries Dr. Rufus Smith.............	126
Their family record	127
3 Fanny Smith and Martin G. Black and family.........	127–132
3 Dr. Charles Smith and family........................	132–134
3 William Coates Smith and family........	134–135
3 Mary E. and Matilda Smith...........................	135
3 Edward B. Smith and family....	135–136
3 Ruth R. Smith and William B. Chandler and family....	138–139
3 Diana G. Smith and L. P. W. Desbrisay and family....	138–139
Posterity of Elizabeth Dixon and Dr. Rufus Smith.......	139

CONTENTS OF CHAPTER VI.

2 Ruth Dixon marries Thomas Roach....	140
Their family record, and death of Mrs. Roach	140
3 John Roach and family........................... ...	141–143
3 Susan Roach and William Crane and family...........	143–144
3 Jean Roach and Michael Gordon and family...........	145–147
3 Charles D. Roach and family.......................	147–149
3 Thomas Roach, Jr., and family	149
3 Edward Roach and family........................ ...	150
Posterity of Ruth Dixon and Thomas Roach.............	151

CONTENTS OF CHAPTER VII.

2 Martha Dixon marries Rev. Benjamin Wilson........ .. 152
Their family record and death of Mr. Wilson........... 153
3 Susanna Wilson and James Sayre and family... 153–155
3 Mary E. Wilson and Doctor Charles Smith............. 155
3 Martha Wilson and Andrew Weldon and family 155–161
3 Jane Ruth Wilson and William P. Sayre and family.... 161–162
3 Fanny B. Wilson and Rev. M. Pickles and family...... 163–165
3 Louisa Ann Wilson and James Harris and family...... 165–166
3 Charles Wilson and family........................... 167–168
3 H. Caroline Wilson and James Potter................. 168
Posterity of Martha Dixon and B. Wilson........ 168

CONTENTS OF CHAPTER VIII.

2 Edward Dixon and Mary Smith married..:............. 169
Their family register................................. 169
3 Charles Dixon and family........................... 170–174
3 Edwin Dixon and family 174–179
3 Elizabeth Dixon and James Chubbuck and family 179–180
3 Jane B. Dixon and David Lyons and family 180–182
3 John E. Dixon and family........ 182–183
3 George Smith Dixon killed........ 183
3 William Coates Dixon and family 183–186
3 Rufus Smith Dixon and family 186–187
3 James D. Dixon and family....... 187–189
Posterity of Edward Dixon and Mary Smith............. 189

CONTENTS OF CHAPTER IX.

2 William Coates Dixon marries Matilda Beckwith...... 190
Their Family Register.... 190–191
Death of Mr. and Mrs. Dixon...................... . 191
3 Horatio Edward Dixon and family................. 191
3 Mary A. Dixon......... 191
3 Caroline Lavinia Dixon and John Smith.............. 191
3 John Steadman Dixon and family. 192
3 William James Dixon and family... 192
Posterity of William Coates Dixon 193
Table of Posterity of Charles and Susanna Dixon....... 194
Conclusion................................. 195

www.ingramcontent.com/pod-product-compliance
Lightning Source LLC
Chambersburg PA
CBHW021731220426
43662CB00008B/793